# HEAL YOUR KNEES

# HEAL YOUR KNEES

## How to Prevent Knee Surgery & What to Do If You Need It

**Robert Klapper, M.D., and Lynda Huey**

M. Evans and Company, Inc.
Lanham • New York • Boulder • Toronto • Plymouth, UK

This M. Evans paperback edition of *Heal Your Knees* is an original publication. It is published by arrangement with the author.

Published by M. Evans
An imprint of The Rowman & Littlefield Publishing Group, Inc.
4501 Forbes Boulevard, Suite 200, Lanham, Maryland 20706

Estover Road
Plymouth PL6 7PY
United Kingdom

Distributed by NATIONAL BOOK NETWORK

The hardback edition of this book was previously cataloged by the Library of Congress as follows:

Klapper, Robert.
    Heal your knees : how to prevent knee surgery and what to do if you need it / Robert Klapper and Lynda Huey.
        p. cm.
    1. Knee—Surgery—Popular works. 2. Knee—Care and hygiene—Popular works. 3. Knee—Diseases—Treatment—Popular works. I. Huey, Lynda. II. Title.
    RD561.K537 2004
    617.5'82044—dc22
                                                                    2004003177
        ISBN-13  978-1-59077-124-2 (pbk. : alk. paper)
        ISBN-10  0-1-59077-124-9 (pbk. : alk. paper)

⊗™ The paper used in this publication meets the minimum requirements of American National Standard for Information Sciences—Permanence of Paper for Printed Library Materials, ANSI/NISO Z39.48-1992.

Manufactured in the United States of America.

For Ellen and Michele Klapper

For Robert and Glenn Margaret Huey

And our friends Roxie and Pepper

And in memory of Wilt Chamberlain,
who started this fine collaboration

# CONTENTS

# ACKNOWLEDGMENTS

The following people contributed to the success of this book:

CompletePT's clinical director, Tanya Moran-Dougherty, MPT, contributed the land exercises in Chapters 1 and 11. She oversaw the shooting of the land exercise photos and helped readers design their own programs in Chapters 8 and 14. Every day she leads CompletePT Pool & Land Physical Therapy with fierce dedication and boundless good cheer.

LeRoy Perry, Jr., D.C., a pioneer in sports medicine and aquatic therapy, has been an inspiration to the authors. Dr. Perry guided Lynda Huey into the water and has provided a solid base of support for her aquatic therapy career.

Orthopedic surgeon Robert Kerlan, M.D., of the Kerlan-Jobe Orthopedic Clinic, inspired Dr. Klapper to do his part in demystifying medicine for the lay public.

The following surgeons at the Hospital for Special Surgery in New York instructed Dr. Klapper in the field of knee surgery: John Insall, M.D., Chit Ranawat, M.D., Russell Warren, M.D., Larry Dorr, M.D., Kelly Vince, M.D., Thomas Sculco, M.D., and Ed McPherson, M.D.

CompletePT's Pool Director, Pattie O'Leary, B.S., PTA, added details and insight to Chapters 10 and 14 and assisted at the pool photo shoot. For eleven years she has been a shining pool goddess at the heart of our successful program.

Author Zan Knudson added insight and ideas throughout the book.

Agent Jane Jordan-Browne helped nurture Lynda Huey's publishing career. She sold three of Lynda's books, found editor PJ Dempsey for this book, then left us, too quickly and too soon, at the age of seventy-one.

Rodger Klein took the underwater and topside pool photos; he also taught Lynda Huey about digital photography and what's possible after the shot has been taken.

Lora Fremont generously allowed us to shoot photos in her pool.

Robert Reiff shot the cover photo, took the land exercise photos, and freely offered advice regarding artwork in the book.

Model LaReine Chabut gracefully posed all the exercise shots.

Jane Sibley-Hasle assisted at all of the photo shoots.

Major Michael Harris of the United States Army Reserves did the medical illustrations.

David Ryer of Moonlight Design created the charts on pages 75, 76, and 151.

Bridget Failner, R.N., head of the Joint Replacement Center at Cedars-Sinai Hospital, provided much of the information in Chapter 13.

Douglas H. Brown, M.D., of Landmark Imaging, schooled us in the new digital-imaging studies and offered details and correct phrasing for Chapter 6, so we could present the new material clearly and accurately.

Tanya Moran-Dougherty, MPT; Pattie O'Leary, B.S., PTA; Jane Sibley-Hasle; Sal Camancho; John Koegel, P.T.; Miranda Mooneyham; Mickie Eng; and Bethany Wright kept CompletePT and Huey's Athletic Network running during Lynda Huey's book-writing absences.

Mark Frantz, Dr. Klapper's X-ray technician, gathered X rays and surgical photos for Chapters 6 and 12.

Bibi Vabrey, Dr. Klapper's office manager, contributed the material in Chapter 5 on identifying emergencies and on forming positive relationships with the doctor's staff.

Adriana Iturrios, Cristina Esparza, Vivian Arango, Adelle Baumgard, and Marion Dillon in Dr. Klapper's office all lent their invaluable assistance whenever needed.

Robby, Ellen, and Michelle Klapper provided Lynda Huey with a writing sanctuary in Ventura, California; David and Denise Fleetham did likewise in Olinda, Maui; and Yogananda did the same at his Self-Realization Fellowship Retreat in Encinitas, California.

Gary Ochman; John Buch; Nick Lozica, M.S., P.T.; Pat Connolly; and Charles Kuntzleman offered their athletic experience and suggestions to Chapter 4.

Mike Shapow, P.T., contributed the astronaut and bear analogies in Chapter 11.

Gary Gagliardi, D.C., gave input in Chapter 7 regarding the use of chiropractic in resolving knee problems.

Ben Hasle offered Lynda Huey a clear mind and listening ear during the whole process.

# PREFACE

Recently a sculptor in Italy told me, "They say when you reach the point of being a master sculptor that you hit with the hammer to the beat of your heart." That's the epitome of being at one with your work—having it be in tune to the beat of your own heart. And that's what I aim for every day as I work either in my vocation as an orthopedic surgeon or in my avocation as a sculptor.

As an art history student at Columbia in the 1970s, I was immediately enamored with Michelangelo's works, but going to medical school delayed my artistic bent. Then, in the late 1990s, I rented studio space in Italy each summer, and, using stones from Michelangelo's quarry at Carrara, began creating my own versions of his best works. Recently I entered my "pieta" into an artists' competition held by the American Academy of Orthopedic Surgeons and was thrilled to have it win the President's Award. My passion for sculpting has grown, especially as I've seen the similarities with my surgical work. I feel the same excitement going to the studio to sculpt as I feel going to the operating room. I'm fully aware that I get to operate on anatomy made by God, and it's a privilege I take very seriously. But I suspect I'm an unusual surgeon in that I try to keep my patients *out* of the operating room.

It's my belief from seeing thousands of patients over the last fifteen years that the best non-surgical approach for joint pain is the water. There's magic in the water on levels we can understand—the weightlessness, the resistance, and the nurturing effect of its warmth—but there are undoubtedly mechanisms at work beyond our understanding involving the balance required in the water and the biofeedback from the water touching the skin. Some of the benefits derived from my patients in the pool are inexplicable at this time, but we know they exist, and we know that's why Lynda Huey and I pursue this collaboration and why it works.

When patients go to the pool, I tell them they are headed toward a win-win situation. They may win after two months of diligent work in the pool by preventing knee surgery altogether. These people win heavily by remaining holistic, getting better without medicine, without shots, without surgery. But even if the architectural damage to the knee is so severe that surgery is inescapable, the second level of win is that they will have prepared for the rigors of surgery and their recovery will be much easier than those people who face surgery without prior rehab exercises. My belief in such "prehab," as rehab prior to surgery is called, has grown stronger in the years since Lynda Huey and I published our first book, *Heal Your Hips*, in 1999. These days, few people enter my operating room who aren't fully prepared for surgery from a month or longer in the pool.

In writing our first book, Lynda and I saw that other books about hip problems weren't available for the lay public. Our mission statement on that book was broad: to educate readers about the anatomy of the hip and bring them up to speed so they could understand sophisticated hip problems. We took our readers into the operating room so they could clearly understand the process of hip implant surgery, or, if they were a candidate for the minimally-invasive hip arthroscopy, so we could explain that procedure.

When it comes to the knee, however, we recognized we wouldn't have the only book on knees on the bookstore shelves. With this book we could highlight the introductory information and move on to other subjects near and dear to my heart, such as how to stop hurting the knees in workouts and how to plan a specific postsurgical rehab program. Our surgery chapter this time isn't an explanation of what happens in the operating room. Instead it is a series of case studies that we feel better serve our readers.

I like to be surrounded in my professional life with people who have a passion for their work, who have been drawn to "a calling" rather than a job or a career. Lynda Huey and I resonate to that same sense of calling, so neither of us is surprised that our combined work continues to grow almost as if it has a life of its own.

—ROBERT KLAPPER, M.D.
*Beverly Hills, California*

If I could have looked into my future when I was twenty-five years old to see that I would spend dozens of years in swimming pools for my life's work, nothing would have surprised me more. I was a serious non-water athlete during my youth and had been told by my track coaches, "Don't go swimming. It uses *different muscles* than running." How absurd! I was one of the first to learn, along with my first crop of Olympic guinea pigs—Jeannette Bolden, Al Joyner, Valerie Brisco, Florence Griffith Joyner, Andre Phillips, Diane Dixon, Willie Banks, Mike Powell, Jackie Joyner-Kersee, Gail Devers, Kim Gallagher, Carole Lewis, and many others—that running in the pool was the best way to retain world-class fitness while injuries healed. During the 1980s, we used Dr. LeRoy Perry's pool at the

International Sportsmedicine Institute, where I was his athletic director and where his pioneering presence in hydrotherapy guided me to my true calling.

My years of competing and coaching led to a private training business, Huey's Athletic Network, which specialized in water rehabilitation. I was the only show in town—in Los Angeles, that is. Great results with star athletes drew headlines, so soon I had to hire other professionals to help handle the growing demand. Ten years later, physical therapists discovered the beauty of water exercise and decided to claim it for themselves. Thankfully, a physical therapist claimed me, too, and I learned the ropes of managing a physical therapy company. I flew all over the United States, western Europe, South America, and Australia teaching my water rehab program to hundreds of physical therapists as the understanding of water's benefits spread. In 1999, my story came full circle as I returned to Dr. Perry's newly-renovated pool and gym with my own growing company, CompletePT Pool & Land Physical Therapy.

Athletic friends from my youth often say to me, "How smart you were to have been in the water all these years." They've continued to run and play tennis, basketball, and beach volleyball. Now, as we all hit our 50s and 60s with the rest of the baby boomers, they are paying the price for their abusive sports—aching and dysfunctioning joints. A former tennis player gave up most of his game because of knee pain; he bicycles instead. A basketball player now plays paddle tennis three days a week at Venice Beach. A beach volleyball player became a devotee of pool workouts and now mixes them in with just a sprinkling of his usual beach activities. And most of my running friends are admitting they don't enjoy pounding the pavement anymore because of back, hip, knee, or foot pain; they are turning to walking or hiking. In essence, we're all "downsizing" our athletic lives. In my case, there hasn't been much change since I've been using pool workouts as the basis of my life-long fitness program for the past twenty years. I've always loved sharing my Waterpower Workout with anyone who was interested, and that group seems to be growing.

Dr. Robert Klapper is such a believer in my pool program that it awes me. Of course I know water works, but to have such a well-respected orthopedic surgeon sing my praises daily to our mutual patients seems quite extraordinary to me. Yes, ours has been a fine collaboration. He has granted me access to his operating room to see first-hand what I have to help rehab. He has opened his energetic mind and let me glean many of his basic philosophies about preventing surgeries. And he has struggled with me to articulate the "magic" that exists in water, which neither of us has yet been able to pinpoint.

Our first book together, *Heal Your Hips*, and our related website, www.hiphelp.com, continue to draw hundreds of patients to his office and my pool program. Ever since that book was published in 1999, patients have asked us, "When are you going to do a knee book?" We've offered people the hip book as well as my book, *The Complete Waterpower Workout Book*, published in 1993, but we knew we'd eventually have to write our knee book. This time, because I oversee a combined pool and land physical-therapy program, I asked my clinical director, Tanya Moran-Dougherty, MPT, to contribute the land exercises to this book, which appear in Chapters 1 and 11. Then, in her wisdom, she asked, "How will patients know what to do and when?" None of the other knee books on the market offer true guidance in that regard. We spent an extra month putting together the non-surgical guidelines in Chapter 8 and the postsurgical guidelines in Chapter 14 so that our readers will have access to our years of experience in leading patients carefully through our programs. Our hope is that we can reach the thousands of people in knee pain who are confused and need guidance in helping themselves to prevent knee surgery—or, if necessary, recovering quickly from it.

—LYNDA HUEY
*Santa Monica, California*

# 1 TEN MINUTES IN WATER, TEN MINUTES ON LAND

*With Tanya Moran-Dougherty, MPT*

Your knee hurts, and you don't know what to do about it.

You've just come home from a long walk or run and suddenly discover a sharp, stabbing pain. Or you've felt an intermittent, deep pain in your knee when you've played basketball for the past few weeks. Or maybe your knee has been hurting off and on for months, no matter what you've been doing: going up and down stairs, walking, standing, or sitting. You sense you've lost your mobility, your ability to move easily through your daily life. And pain keeps you awake at night.

You may have developed an abnormal gait. You may limp briefly when first rising from a chair or getting out of your car. Or you may limp with every step. Your friends may point this out to you even though you no longer can feel how you're quickly shifting your weight from the sore knee onto the stronger one.

Or years ago you were told that you have a "knee condition" that would "catch up with you" later in life. Now you fear your pain will go on forever.

Whether your knee pain is a complete surprise, a growing concern, or a problem you knew was bound to happen, **you want relief**: you want less pain and easier, smoother movements. You don't want to harm your knee further, but you aren't sure how to protect it. You **do know** you have to exercise in order to regain or maintain your strength and optimum mobility, but you need guidance. You want to learn the safest way to set goals to **heal your knees.**

In years past, your previous physical goals may have been to walk more miles, to score more points, to run a faster race, to win more sets of tennis, or to ski a higher mountain. Or, because you've been sedentary for years, you've had no physical goals. In either case, you now must train to be pain-free: to recognize quickly the first signals of pain, to adapt your lifestyle to protect and nurture your knees, and always to move toward increasing strength and capability. As your knee improves, you will be diminishing your knee pain—a true athletic challenge.

Here's the proven best way to start. Go to your nearest swimming pool and do the ten-minute program that follows. The pain relief and sense of healing you'll feel will be forever worth the effort of traveling to the water. This will be the day you begin your "come back"—your first step on the road to knee fitness.

## TEN-MINUTE POOL PROGRAM

Copy the box on the next page, laminate it and take it to the pool with you. Place it poolside and follow the order of the exercises. Do each exercise for one minute.

While doing the exercises, focus on the differing capabilities of your left and right  knees. Does one knee bend more than the other? Does one knee straighten more easily? Notice whether you take a longer stride with one leg than with the other or whether you feel stronger while weight-bearing on one knee than the other.

**Ten-Minute Pool Program**

Exercise 1. Walking forward, backward, and sideways

Exercise 2. Marching

Exercise 3. Hamstring Stretch

Exercise 4. Back Flutter Kicks

Exercise 5. Bicycle Kicks

Exercise 6. Quad Extensions

Exercise 7. Hamstring Curls

Exercise 8. Squats

## EXERCISE 1. SHALLOW WATER WALKING WARM-UP

Spend three minutes on this exercise—one minute walking forward, one backward, and one sideways. Walk forward and backward across the pool in **chest-deep water** until you've become accustomed to the water temperature. Even if you limp on land, aim toward a normal gait in the water. Next, walk sideways, first leading with one leg, then the other leg.

**KNEE NOISE WITHOUT PAIN IS INSIGNIFICANT**

Even if your knees pop and crunch every time you bend them, that's nothing to worry about unless you also have associated pain. Just as when you crack your knuckles, that noise doesn't mean your fingers are having trouble; neither is a noisy knee without pain a sign of trouble.

## EXERCISE 2. MARCHING

Begin marching by lifting a knee to ninety degrees as shown in photo 1-2 or as high as you can lift without feeling increased knee pain. Lean forward and take a step, then lift the other knee to a similar position.

If you feel pain in your sore knee, try these modifications: first move to deeper water, then try moving more slowly. Or if pain persists, don't lift your knee as high. Pay attention to the directions your knees are pointing while

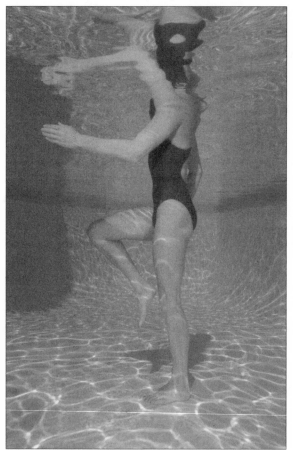

you march—both knees should point straight forward, not out to the sides or across the midline of your body. Bend your arms in opposition to your bent knees: your right arm should move in time with your left knee, and your left arm should move with your right knee.

Notice if both knees are lifting to the same height and bending equally. Aim toward symmetry in all your movements; that is, use both sides of your body equally, particularly both knees.

1-2 Marching

## EXERCISE 3. HAMSTRING STRETCH

Hold the side of the pool with both hands. Place your left foot, toes up, against the pool wall, as shown in photo 1-3. Keep your neck, shoulders, arms, and back relaxed throughout the exercise. Gently straighten your left knee as far as you can while you breathe deeply and slowly five times (approximately thirty seconds). If this is too difficult or causes too much pain, place your foot lower on the pool wall or onto a low step in the pool.

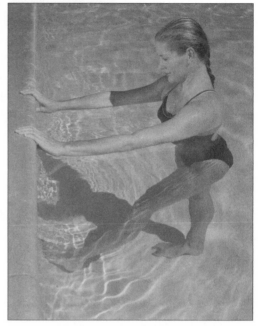

**1-3** Hamstring stretch

**LISTEN TO YOUR BODY**

As you position yourself for these exercises, you might feel the urge to move your leg or body in a way that isn't part of the program. That's your body talking to you. Try to follow its guidance. For example, if you feel like flexing and pointing your foot or making circles at the ankle to relax your calf muscles, do it. Intuitive knowledge surfaces in the water, so pay attention to what you're feeling and what movements your body asks of you. You will learn to read your body more precisely by paying attention to it in the water.

## EXERCISE 4. BACK FLUTTER KICKS

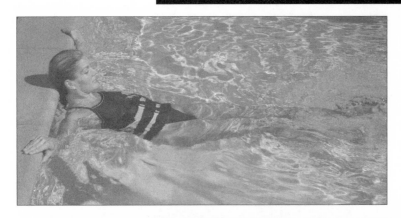

Brace yourself with your back to the pool wall and your arms on the edge of the pool or on the pool's gutter. Lift your hips and legs and begin shallow flutter kicks with straight legs (See photo 1-4).

1-4 Back flutter kicks

## EXERCISE 5. BICYCLE KICKS

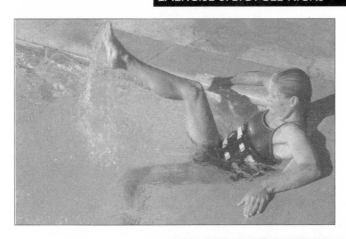

Continue bracing yourself at the side of the pool. Bend your knees and begin kicking in a bicycling movement, as shown in photo 1-5. Notice that a corner can be used for improved comfort during this exercise.

1-5 Bicyle Kick

## EXERCISE 6. QUAD EXTENSIONS

Quad extensions are exercises that use the quadriceps muscles, located on the front of your thighs, to extend your knee. To do these, hold your left knee in front of you, foot dangling toward the pool bottom (See photo 1-6A). Gently straighten your leg (See photo 1-6B), then bend it again to the starting position. If you feel pain, slow the movement, lower the knee, or do both.

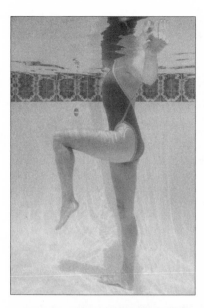

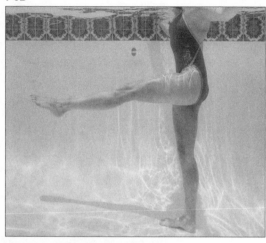

**1-6A** Quad Extensions

**1-6B**

## EXERCISE 7. HAMSTRING CURLS

Hamstring curls use your hamstring muscles, located on the back of your thighs, to bend your knees. Start with your knees together, feet together on the bottom of the pool. Keep your knees together as you lift your left heel toward the left buttock (See photo 1-7), then push your foot back to the pool bottom. Lift up and push down with equal force, reaching for full flexion (bending) and extension (straightening).

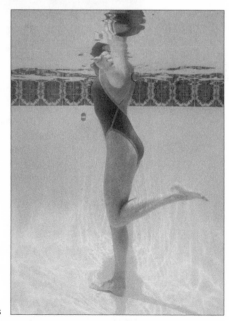

**1-7** Hamstring Curls

## EXERCISE 8. SQUATS

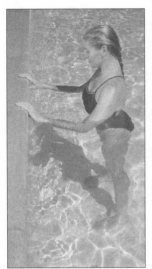

**1-8A** Squats

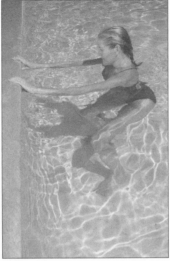

**1-8B**

Face the side of the pool in chest-deep water, with your feet parallel and shoulder-width apart. Grasp the side of the pool with both hands (See photo 1-8A). Keep your back straight and slowly bend both knees until your chin touches the water, as shown in Photo 1-8B. At the lowest point in your squat, your heels will probably lift away from the pool bottom.

---

**WATER WORKS!**

Here's how water works: As soon as you step into the pool, you've eliminated the weightbearing cause of your pain. Once you've taken a "load" off of your sore knee, you move it more easily through its range of motion against the smooth resistance of the water. Your knee gets stronger. In fact, no matter which direction you move in water—up, down, forward, backward, bending, or straightening— you encounter water's three-dimensional resistance, and you continue strengthening the muscles surrounding your knee.

---

You'll probably discover that your whole body feels refreshed and you don't want to get out of the pool after only ten minutes. You move more easily in the water, and the pain in your knee has diminished. But don't overdo this first pool session. Stop before you encounter fatigue or pain. You can always return to the water, and it will become your most forgiving friend.

   Yet you can't live your life in a pool. You need your knee to function well on land so you can perform the movements of your daily life. Use the program that follows.

## TEN-MINUTE LAND PROGRAM

When you return from the pool, find a carpeted space where you can comfortably perform these exercises. You'll need a straight-backed, stable chair for Exercises 12 and 13. Do the exercises with the stronger knee first, then try them with the more affected knee. If you feel an increase in knee pain, slow your movements, narrow your range of motion, or both. If pain persists, skip that exercise and move on to the next.

### EXERCISE 9. HEEL SLIDES

Sit erect with a towel or strap wrapped around the ball of your foot and grasp both ends, as shown in photo 1-9A. Slowly bend your knee and use the towel to help slide your heel toward your buttocks (see photo 1-9B). Bend your knee as much as possible without increasing your pain, then return to the starting position. Do ten repetitions on this side, then repeat on the other side, moving slowly and staying in this knee's pain-free range of motion. Compare the amount of pain-free movement you have in each knee.

**1-9A** Heel slides

**1-9B**

## EXERCISE 10. QUAD SETS

Sit erect with both legs straight in front of you, your hands behind you for balance. Roll a towel and place it under your stronger knee (see photo 1-10). Keep your toes pulled back toward your head. Tighten your quadriceps muscles while pushing the back of your knee into the towel. You should see your kneecap move slightly toward your hip if you perform this exercise correctly. Hold for a count of six, and then slowly release. Do ten reps on this side, then repeat on the other side. Compare how similarly or differently the two knees feel and function. Notice if one leg is stronger than the other.

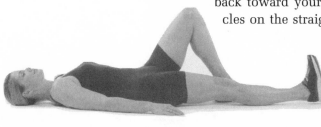

**1-10** Quad sets

## EXERCISE 11. STRAIGHT-LEG RAISES

Lie on the floor, as shown in photo 1-11A, with one knee bent and the other leg straight in front of you with the toes pulled back toward your body. Tighten your thigh muscles on the straight leg and slowly lift it straight up to the position shown in photo 1-11B. When you lower the leg, make sure your calf muscles touch the floor first, not your heel. If your heel touches first, you've bent your knee. Try again, keeping your leg straight. Do ten straight-leg raises on each side.

**1-11A** Straight-leg raises

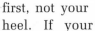

**1-11B**

## EXERCISE 12. QUADRICEPS EXTENSION

Sit in a stable chair as shown in photo 1-12A. Lift one foot, straightening your knee as fully as you can without increasing your pain (see photo 1-12B). Slowly lower the foot, bending the knee to the starting position. **Stay in your pain-free range of motion.** This means you should do only the portion of the movement that doesn't cause you pain. Do ten repetitions. Rest, then repeat on the other leg.

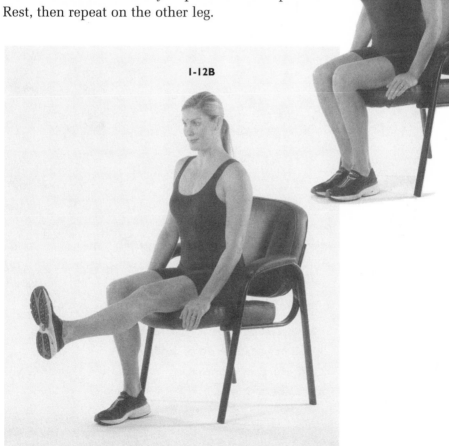

**1-12A**
Quadriceps extension

**1-12B**

## EXERCISE 13. HAMSTRING CURLS

**Do this exercise *only* with the affected knee while standing on your stronger leg.**

Stand, holding the back of a chair or a table for balance. Bend your affected knee by bringing your heel toward your buttocks (see photo 1-13). Don't let your working knee drift forward—it should stay in line with your standing knee. Focus on your hamstring muscles as they lift and lower your heel. Do ten repetitions.

**1-13**
Hamstring curls

After your ten minutes in water and ten minutes on land, you probably feel for yourself that your knee is moving more easily, less painfully. You have just discovered some important truths:

- Water exercises allow you to perform movements that would be painful to do on land.
- Land exercises more nearly duplicate the challenges you must face in daily life.
- Movement heals.

# 2 FIT KNEES

It will be tempting to turn past these technical chapters and go directly to the pleasurable workouts that follow. But anyone with knee pain or limitation of movement will find it useful to understand how knees "work," and, if they don't work, why. Learning more about the structure of your knees will turn you into an educated patient who can discriminate between minor pains that can be treated at home and more significant pains that may require seeking help from a doctor, physical therapist, or others. You will be able to ask careful questions that will demystify knee function, help allay your concerns, and enable you take an integral part in your healing.

The knee is not a simple hinge joint that bends and straightens. Rather, it is **probably the most complicated joint in the body:** It contains three separate and equally important joints which, working together, bend, straighten, and also permit the limited rotation needed to do a full squat.

The knee joint is where the femur (thigh bone) attaches to the two bones of the lower leg—the tibia (shin bone) and the fibula, which is the smaller bone on the

**2-1A&B**
Part A shows the boney anatomy of a right knee from the front, in which can be seen the medial and lateral joint compartments.

Part B is a side view of a left knee showing the patella in its groove along the front of the femur.

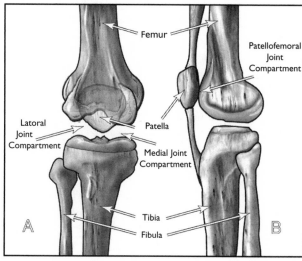

Femur

Patellofemoral Joint Compartment

Latoral Joint Compartment

Patella

Medial Joint Compartment

Tibia

Fibula

A

B

side (see illustration 2-1, Part A). The medial, or inner compartment of the joint, is where your two knees touch each other when you put your legs together. There's an entirely separate lateral compartment to the knee, which you can locate when you reach down to touch the outsides of your knees. The third part of the knee joint is the patellofemoral joint, where the cartilage behind the kneecap meets the groove in the femur (see illustration 2-1, Part B.) When you flex (bend) and extend (straighten) your knee, the patella glides through a groove in the femur called the trochlea.

This beautiful job of engineering, this knee joint, is made stable through its entire range of movement—from full flexion to full extension—by its four key supporting ligaments. The medial collateral ligament (MCL) runs from the femur to the tibia down the inside border of the knee and limits the sideways motion of the knee (see illustration 2-2, Part A.) The lateral collateral ligament (LCL) runs down the outside border of the knee and limits sideways motion in the opposite direction. Two cruciate ligaments cross each other through the middle of the joint. (*Cruciate* in Latin means "cross.") One goes in front, the anterior cruciate ligament (ACL), and the other goes in back, the posterior cruciate ligament (PCL) (see illustration 2-2, Part B). The cruciates serve a dual purpose: they stabilize the knee, front to back, and protect it during rotation.

Two different types of cartilage cushion the knee joint: the hyaline cartilage and the meniscus cartilage. Like all joints, the knee has hyaline or articular cartilage covering the ends of the bones. This thin smooth layer covers the ends of all bones in the body and protects bones from impact forces.

**2-2 A&B**
Part A is a front view of a knee showing its stabilizing ligaments.

Part B is a side view of the knee's ligament.

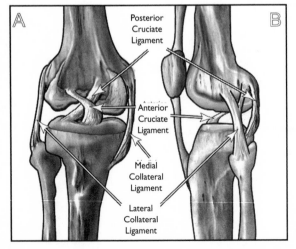

Posterior Cruciate Ligament

Anterior Cruciate Ligament

Medial Collateral Ligament

Lateral Collateral Ligament

Unlike the other joints, the knee has a disk-shaped meniscus cushion in each of the lateral and medial compartments to provide extra shock absorption between the femur and the tibia. These mensici are made of rubbery fibrocartilage, the same material found in your ear and nose. The periphery of the medial meniscus is directly attached to the deep structures of the MCL, so whenever you have a disruption of the MCL, it can cause an injury to the meniscus and vice versa. The lateral meniscus has a tendon that goes through the center of it, making its circulation and nourishment more at risk than that of the medial meniscus. The popliteal tendon at the center of the lateral meniscus creates a nonvascular hole, which complicates any meniscal tears or surgeries in that area (see illustration 2-3, Part A).

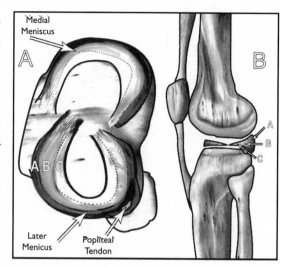

**2-3 A&B**
Part A is an overhead view of the three zones of the meniscus.

Part B:
A is the the red-red zone.
B is the red-white zone.
C is the white-white zone.

Fit knees have hyaline cartilage that functions so smoothly you don't feel any friction as you move. To understand more clearly the smooth movement made possible by the cartilage in your knees, go to your freezer and take out two ice cubes. Wet them and rub them against each other. Feel how slippery they are. There is almost no friction as one glides across the surface of the other. Now try to visualize a fit knee joint. The surfaces of that joint are even more slippery than the ice cubes. As the knee bends, straightens, and slightly rotates, the contact between the various sections of the joint is so delicate that the friction—the amount that they rub together—is less than that of your two ice cubes.

Hyaline cartilage does not have a blood supply. Rather, it receives its nourishment from a flow of fluids, behaving almost like a sponge. You squeeze the sponge and water is pushed out; you release the sponge, and it sucks up water. Similarly, you take a step and put weight on your knee, and joint fluid is squeezed out of the hyaline cartilage. When you lift your leg to take another step, the joint fluid rushes back into the cartilage. The nourishing fluids move in and out as your cartilage responds to the changing forces exerted on your knee joint.

Nourishment of the meniscus is even more fascinating. The meniscus is divided into three zones, each of which has its own form of nourishment. In illustration 2-3, Part B, you can see the side view of the meniscus, showing its wedge-shaped, gradual change in thickness. The periphery is completely, intimately attached to the joint capsule. Blood vessels from the capsule enter the outer one-third of the meniscus and supply all its nutrients. This portion of the meniscus is known as the "red-red zone" because it is fed by a blood supply. The red-red section is the thickest part of the meniscus. The middle third of the meniscus is called the "red-white zone" because half of its nourishment comes from blood circulation and half comes from the sponge-like system of the joint fluids. The inner one-third, the portion of the meniscus closest to the center of the joint, is called the "white-white zone" and is the thinnest part of the wedge-shaped meniscus tissue. It depends solely on joint fluid for its nourishment.

The tough fibers and ligaments that encase the knee joint are called the joint capsule. These connective tissues envelope the joint, holding it together. A pre-patella bursal sac in front of the kneecap is filled with fluid and is situated on the kneecap's surface where pressure is applied when you kneel. This cushioning relieves that  pressure and also prevents friction.

All joints are lined with a synovial membrane that produces synovial fluid. Synovial fluid is a transparent alkaline fluid resembling egg white that lubricates and feeds cartilage surfaces. This joint fluid inside the knee may hold the key to the function of knee joints. The joint fluid has been largely overlooked by orthopedists in the past but is now a factor under study in problem knees. Just as a muscle frays and degenerates, just as our skin loses elasticity, so does the fluid within the knee begin to degenerate.

Compare joint fluid in your knee with motor oil in the cylinders of your car. The acidity changes over time, the viscosity or thickness of the oil changes, and those changes decrease the oil's ability to do its job. Similarly, joint fluid degenerates with time, becoming more acidic and therefore less helpful as a lubricant. In fact, it can begin to harm the surface of the cartilage. We suspect there are dozens of functions we have yet to discover that are performed by joint fluid, so any decrease in its quality would diminish those functions.

---

**THE CHICKEN OR THE EGG?**

Researchers don't yet know which comes first: does arthritis begin breaking down the cartilage in the joint, causing the joint fluid to react, or does decaying fluid trigger the cartilage damage of arthritis? Whoever answers this question will win a Nobel Prize! If the joint fluid proves to be the trigger, a synthesized fluid might be developed that could stop the advancement of arthritis.                                          —ROBERT KLAPPER, M.D.

---

The kneecap, a sesamoid bone, may be the most unusual feature of the knee. We've all learned about a fulcrum, either through using a jack to change a tire or by trying to move something heavy like a refrigerator. If you stand beside the refrigerator and try to lift it, you find you can't because it's too heavy. But if you take a crowbar and a simple piece of wood to use as a fulcrum, you can lift the refrig-

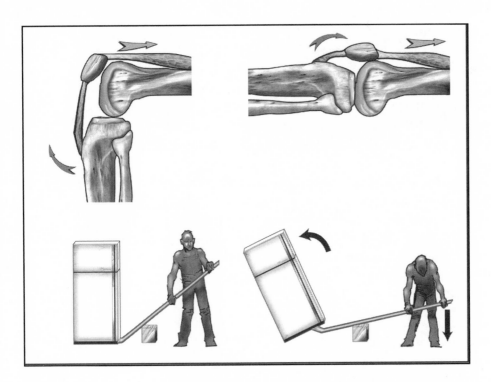

**2-4**

The patella is a sesamoid bone that acts as a fulcrum for the knee, allowing the quadriceps to generate great power as they straighten the knee.

erator with ease (see illustration 2-4). The fulcrum and the lever arm create a mechanical advantage, magnifying your strength to perform the work. Similarly, our knees have a fulcrum—the knee cap. The quad muscle is the crowbar, the patella is the fulcrum, and the quad's attachment to the tibial tubercle is the refrigerator. The result of lifting the refrigerator is the straightening of your knee. The quad muscle goes up and over the patella, giving a mechanical advantage to the entire quadriceps mechanism. A leg with a patella can exert much greater strength than a leg that has lost its patella to injury. The patella is such a critical player in knee function that it truly is a key to your body's mobility and power.

# THE MUSCLES THAT MOVE THE KNEE

Any time a muscle crosses a joint, it will have an effect on that joint. Muscles located in the thighs and calves cross the knee joint to control movement at the knee. Tendons attach those muscles to the bones on both sides of the joint. Illustrations 2-5, Part A, and 2-5, Part B show the muscles and tendons that move the knee. The quadriceps flex (bend) the hip and extend (straighten) the knee. The hamstrings flex (bend) the knee and extend (straighten) the hip. While the quads and hamstrings are the primary movers of the knee, other muscles cross the knee joint and therefore are either secondary movers or stabilizers. For example, the adductor muscles on the insides of the thighs work in combination with the quads to help kick a soccer ball across the front of the body. (See illustration 3-4 on page 47.) The

**2-5 A&B**
In Part A, a front view of the knee, the quadriceps muscles run down the front of the thigh, and when they conract, they extend (straighten) the knee. In Part B, a side view of the knee, the hamstrings run down the back of the thigh and the gastrocnemius runs down the back of the calf—both muscle groups flex (bend) the knee.

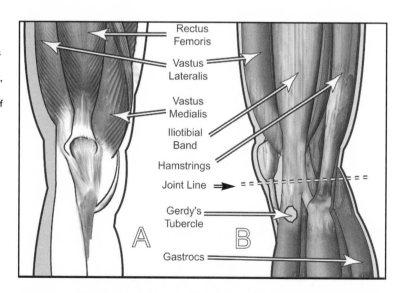

Rectus Femoris

Vastus Lateralis

Vastus Medialis

Iliotibial Band

Hamstrings

Joint Line

Gerdy's Tubercle

Gastrocs

A   B

abductor muscles and iliotibial band run down the outside of the thigh and assist other combinations of movements that would swing the leg out to the side. The gastrocnemius, anchored at the back of the calf, helps flex the knee.

Other joints of the body, such as the shoulder and the hip, are surrounded with muscles that help protect them and maintain their stability. By contrast, the knee has no muscles padding it, and is quite vulnerable and unprotected. Is it any wonder that injuries happen so often to the knee?

Chapter 3 explains the many things that can go wrong with knees to render them unfit.

# 3 UNFIT KNEES

Once you start to feel pain, instability, or limited movement in your knee, a downward spiral begins. If you've been aware of your knee condition for a while, but have taken no measure to combat it, you may have already entered this Negative Spiral, shown below.

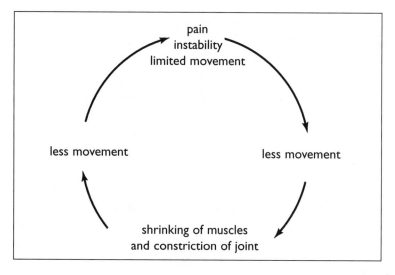

**Negative Spiral**

First you feel pain, instability, or limitation of movement, so you move your knee less often. You sit more each day. You drive your car to places you used to walk, skip your workouts at the gym, even find yourself asking others to walk the dog. Because you are no longer moving your knee joint, it isn't receiving the fluids and nourishment it requires, and it becomes further constricted and inflamed. The muscles begin shrinking, a process called atrophy. Once these muscles start feeling weak, you use them even less, and they atrophy more. The tendons, ligaments, and capsule in and around the knee joint aren't being stretched to their usual length, and they begin to lose their elasticity, becoming brittle and likely to tear. Further, if you alter your gait due to knee pain, you can develop overcompensation injuries in the hip and the lower back.

Here's an analogy that you can apply to your sore knee: imagine you've broken your foot and doctors have put it in a cast so the bones can heal. But they also confine the muscles and tendons of your calf. When the cast comes off weeks later, the X ray looks fine, but your leg is shriveled from disuse. Now you have aches and pains coming from the tissues that were immobilized. The tendons and ligaments weren't stressed, so they weren't lubricated and they lost flexibility. The muscles didn't contract, so they atrophied and lost strength. In the same way, if you stop moving your knee due to pain, you are virtually placing your knee in a cast, and the muscles, ligaments, and tendons around your knee will suffer the same fate as those around the broken foot.

It is indeed a Negative Spiral: lack of movement causes increased soft tissue involvement, which in turn causes more pain, so you move even less.

You want to turn this cycle around, and you can. You can bring the muscles, ligaments, and tendons around your knee back to health, diminish pain, and increase your mobility.

If you've bought this book, you probably already have pain, instability, or limited motion in your knee joint. If you nodded with recognition while reading about the Negative Spiral, you may have already decreased your activity and begun noticing that your knee is getting worse. It's time to learn more about what's going wrong with your knee.

## COMMON CAUSES OF KNEE PROBLEMS

Most joints of the body have ligaments that wrap around the outside of the joint to protect it and offer stability. The knee shares that construction by having two ligaments protecting the outside of the joint. But the knee is also the only joint to have so many structures—two cruciate ligaments and two disk-shaped menisci—inside the actual joint. When sudden forces hit the knee during complex movements that combine flexion, extension, and two planes of rotation, it's not uncommon to see more than one injury happen at the same time.

Your knee may not have suffered a sudden injury but rather have been degenerating over months or years. Here are the most common injuries and degenerative joint conditions.

### Meniscus Tears

As you age, the meniscus weakens and becomes more fragile, just like all the other tissues in your body. Whereas it might have taken a football injury in your youth to tear a meniscus, in your older years it can happen simply from squatting.

The classic presentation of a torn meniscus is a stabbing pain along the knee joint line. To find the joint line, think of your knee as a clock. The 12 o'clock position is at the center of the top of your kneecap (see illustration 3-1 on page 40). The 6 o'clock position, called the inferior pole of the patella, is at

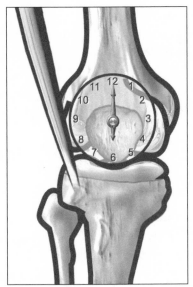

**3-1**
By picturing the face of a clock on your knee, you can perform a self-diagnosis for a torn meniscus.

the bottom of your kneecap. Place your index and middle fingers at the 6 o'clock position, then slide your hand across the joint line to the outside and to the inside. If you have a sharp, stabbing pain on the inner portion, odds are you have a torn medial meniscus. If you feel sharp pain on the outer portion, it's probably a torn lateral meniscus. If your knee pain is above or below the joint line, you probably have an injury that isn't a torn meniscus.

What to do about a meniscus tear depends on the kind of tear, the quality of the meniscus that's left, and on the location of the tear. Meniscus tears are graded by many factors (see illustration 3-2, Parts A–D). Is it a horizontal tear, called a cleavage tear? Is it vertical, called a radial tear? Did the meniscus tear at an angle? Is it a complex tear, which is a combination of all of the others? Where is it located? Is it in the back half of the knee, the posterior horn? Is it in the front half of the knee, the anterior horn? Is it in the middle of the knee?

**3-2**
Part A: A horizontal meniscus tear, called a cleavage tear.
Part B: A vertical meniscus tear, called a radical tear. Part C: A meniscus torn at an angle.
Part D: A complex meniscus tear, which is a combination of all of the other tears.

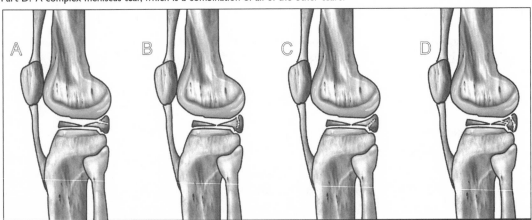

**CHANGING BELIEFS**

Thirty years ago, doctors thought the meniscus was as expendable as the appendix. If there was a tear in a meniscus, surgeons removed the whole thing. What is dogma in one generation turns out to be the opposite in another generation. Who knows? Ten years from now, we may find out people live longer if they keep their appendixes and tonsils.

If a man in his eighties tears a meniscus, it wouldn't make sense to try to repair it, because that would be like trying to put stitches in a Boston cream pie. It wouldn't work. Even if it's an easy, repairable tear, the older patient is best served by trimming away and vacuuming out the torn part of the meniscus and leaving behind as much of the functioning meniscus as possible. But in a younger person, say in her twenties or thirties, we'll try to repair the meniscus rather than remove it. However, it's like real estate: location, location, location. If the tear is in the red-red zone of the meniscus, a repair can be attempted, since this area has enough blood supply to allow subsequent healing. (See illustrations 2-3 on page 31.) When damage occurs in the red-white zone, this **may** be repairable. In the white-white zone, attempts to repair the meniscus with stitches uniformly fail, because there's no blood supply to make viable scar tissue. In that case, the portion of the meniscus that's torn is trimmed out, leaving as much as possible. If the entire meniscus were removed, as doctors used to do routinely, the development of osteoarthritis (see pages 51 to 53) in the joint would be accelerated, because the hyaline cartilage would be at much greater risk, no longer having its extra-protective cushion.

> **BECOME AN EDUCATED PATIENT**
> When your doctor tells you that you have a torn meniscus, it would thrill me for you to be able to respond with this: "Is it in the anterior or posterior horn? Is it a horizontal cleavage tear, a radial tear, or a bucket handle tear? Is it in the red-red, red-white, or white-white zone, and is there a meniscal cyst associated with it?"                        —ROBERT KLAPPER, M.D.

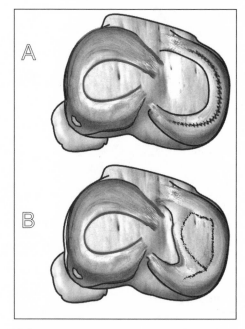

**3-3**
A bucket handle meniscus tear in place (Part A), then flipped out to look like a bucket handle (Part B).

By contrast to the types of meniscus tears previously listed, the bucket handle tear is the extravaganza of all tears, because it is the most extensive. Illustration 3-3, Part A, shows how such a vertical tear runs the entire length of the curved meniscus. Then, once it is displaced and flips out of position (illustration 3-3, Part B), its shape looks like a bucket handle.

If any one of these meniscus tears is severe enough to detach itself from its anchoring site, it can become a free-floating doorstop inside the space between the tibia and the femur. All it takes is to have that piece of cartilage lodge in the right spot, and you've got a locked knee. It's like trying to open a door when the doorstop's there. You can't do it.

People come into my office and say, "I twisted my knee playing baseball. Now I can't bend or straighten it." Or "I twisted it in the kitchen, and now my knee is stuck at a 45-degree angle." By definition, that is a meniscus tear with a displaced fragment. We usually schedule surgery within the next day or two. You can't wait a week.

**ATTENTION HMO USERS!**
If you have a locked knee, don't wait around for a referral to your orthopedist. If you can't get an appointment right away, go to your local emergency room. You'll need to have an MRI and possible surgery within the next day or two at the latest.

Some people have a genetic abnormality of the lateral meniscus called a discoid meniscus. Instead of the usual kidney-shaped meniscus that is thicker on the periphery and thinner at the central portion, a discoid meniscus is flat and fills up the entire surface between the tibia and femur. You would think this would be the ultimate cushion to protect the knee against osteoarthritis, but that turns out not to be the case because the discoid meniscus is thicker than normal, is badly constructed, and is therefore at greater risk of tearing than a normal meniscus. So when a discoid meniscus tears, surgeons are faced with a challenge: trim out the torn portion only, as in a traditional meniscus tear, or go beyond what's torn and try to make a more normal-looking, kidney-shaped meniscus? Going a step further, should it be taken out altogether and have a meniscal transplant from a cadaver? I try to keep things simple. I trim out

**MENISCAL TRANSPLANTS**
There's a saying in medicine: **When you're a hammer, all the world looks like a nail.** Just because you **can** do something doesn't mean that you **should** do it. Meniscal transplants are being done too often these days simply because they've become possible. If your hyaline cartilage has advanced damage, putting in a new meniscus isn't necessarily the correct solution.

what's torn and shape the meniscus as best I can into a normal-looking one. But if the patient persists in having knee trouble, that would be the time to consider a transplant. Few orthopedic surgeons regularly perform meniscal transplants, so do your research to find one with experience.

## Ligament Injuries

When ligaments are injured, the joint is said to have been sprained. Ligament injuries can be mild, with microscopic tears in the fibers, or they can be more severe, with increased amounts of torn fibers and accompanied bleeding. Taking the injury further, the ligament can tear completely, totally disrupting the function of that structure. Each knee ligament requires a different treatment.

The medial collateral ligament (MCL) is vulnerable to blows from the side, such as those often sustained in football or in skiing. In the not too distant past, when you tore an MCL it was recommended that your surgeon make an incision, find the two ends, and either suture or staple them back together. Today we know better. Consider the way your skin heals if you cut it: you stop the bleeding, you bandage it, your body makes a clot that becomes a scab, and a year later you have a line on your skin. You barely remember that you cut yourself. The MCL, being located just beneath the skin, can follow that same healing process. It bleeds, it makes a clot, it organizes the clot, remodels it as necessary, and ultimately heals on its own. Instead of surgically repairing the MCL, we simply put patients in knee braces so they can't create further damage. **If you tore your MCL, you probably won't need surgery.**

The cruciates, however, are a different story. Since they are located inside the knee joint, they are constantly bathed with joint fluid. When the ACL tears, the blood from the torn ligament spills into the joint, and the joint fluid there prevents the bleeding from going to the next step of forming a clot—similar to keeping your hand in  dishwater all day and hoping a skin wound would heal. The joint fluid doesn't allow the bleeding, clotting, and scarring cascade to happen as with the MCL. So this means surgery. We're very good at surgically repairing the ACL ligament, but we don't have such good success repairing the PCL. If you check the literature in orthopedics, you'll find that the PCL's unique anatomy uniformly leads to terrible surgical repair results. Nevertheless, there are plenty of surgeons who will tell you they'll be happy to fix your PCL. Don't let them unless your PCL has debilitated you to the point that walking is difficult. **If you tore your PCL, you'd better get a second and third opinion before undergoing surgery.**

The lateral collateral ligament (LCL) is a combination of both the previous scenarios: sometimes it will heal on its own, and sometimes it won't. Since the main nerve that runs down the leg, the peroneal nerve, is so close to the LCL, operating on this ligament is dangerous. The body is its own best healer, and I like to wait to see if the body can heal it before I recommend surgery. Then, if I must surgically repair an LCL, I remind myself I'm in "Tiger Country": something might come and bite me, such as the artery or the nerve. I have to be extremely careful.

---

**HEAR THE WARNINGS YOUR BODY WHISPERS**

If you've been lucky enough to have suffered only a mild knee sprain with no torn ligaments, take it as a warning. Use the self treatments in Chapter 7 to speed its healing and switch immediately to the nurturing activities in Chapter 4. Don't keep doing your usual workouts. Learn to listen to the warnings your body whispers to you so it won't eventually have to shout at you to be heard.

## Tendon Injuries

Under a microscope, the structure of tendons and ligaments appear very similar. They're both made of collagen, a protein structure that is one of the main elements of many of the body's tissues. The key difference between tendons and ligaments is that tendons attach muscle to bone while ligaments attach bone to bone. Tendons are involved with movement while ligaments are static and involved with stability.

Tendons are generally injured through movement—too much movement too suddenly, causing an acute tendon problem, or too much of the same movement, causing a progressive overuse injury. Tendinitis means inflammation of the tendon. You can create inflammation in any of the tendons near the knee through macro-trauma, a one-time impact or injury, or through micro-trauma, small microscopic tears in the tendon which, if left untreated, can lead to increased pain and dysfunction. Micro-trauma often comes in the form of repetitive exercise such as running, stair climbing, or using a treadmill. Visualize rubbing your fingernail back and forth over a spot on a cotton shirt. If you keep doing it, eventually you'll start to wear a hole in it, just as repetitive exercise does to your tendons.

Three tendons near the knee are often inflamed with tendinitis: the iliotibial band (ITB), the patellar tendon, and the pes anserinus tendon (an attachment of the hamstring to the knee). People who are new to exercise, as well as weekend warriors, often experience any or all of these. Even if you've exercised for years, if you dramatically increase your training, such as in preparation for a first marathon, you may learn about these first hand.

The iliotibial band runs from the hip down the thigh to a spot below the knee that is called Gerdy's tubercle, a bony prominence on the top of the tibia on the lateral side of the knee (see illustration 3-4). You can almost feel Gerdy's tubercle with your fingers where the ITB attaches.

The patellar tendon, just below the kneecap, attaches from the 6 o'clock position of the patella onto the front of the tibia. Runners, hurdlers, jumpers, and volleyball and basketball players often experience patellar tendinitis, which is also called "jumper's knee."

One of the hamstring muscles, the semitendinosis, ends in the pes anserinus tendon. The name of this tendon in Latin means goose's foot, because where the tendon attaches to the medial side of the top of the tibia looks like the webbed foot of a goose. Sprinters and other high-speed competitive athletes often inflame this tendon.

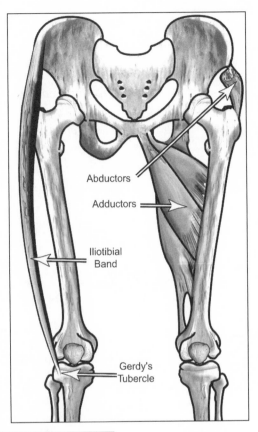

**3-4**

The iliotibial band runs down the side of the thigh and attaches below the knee at Gerdy's tubercle, which can become inflamed with tendinitis.

**SELF DIAGNOSIS**

The classic way you can make a self-diagnosis and reassure yourself that you haven't damaged a meniscus or a ligament is to place your fingers at the 6 o'clock position of your knee (see illustration 3-1 on page 40). Slide your fingers along the joint line of your knee both medially (toward the inside) and laterally (toward the outside). Your fingers obviously aren't an MRI, but they can tell you a lot. If your pain is above or below the joint line, the chances are very good that you have tendinitis rather than a torn meniscus inside the joint.

The next time you drive over a suspension bridge, look at the cables. Five to ten tiny wire cables are wrapped together as a bunch. Each bunch is wrapped and braided with another five or ten bunches. Then that bunch is braided with another five or ten larger bunches for maximum strength. The collagen fibers in your tendons are constructed in the same strong, braided manner. Yet in spite of such strength of the overall tendon, micro-trauma can cause tearing in the tiny fibers in your tendons. That's what tendinitis is: a microscopic tearing of small fibers. When such tears occur, small blood vessels in the tendons break and bleed. The blood that spills into the surrounding tissues becomes an irritant to the nerve endings in that area, causing pain and swelling. Although painful, tendinitis doesn't mean you need surgery. It means you need to stop doing whatever is aggravating the inflamed tendon. You need to let the tendon rest so your body can heal it. Other self-treatments appear in Chapter 7.

---

**DON'T INJECT CORTISONE INTO TENDINITIS**

Cortisone injections are a common cause of ruptured tendons. One of my patients is an ultra-fit, fifty-five-year-old who plays tennis with a friend, who is also his rheumatologist. Over the last few years the rheumatologist gave him six cortisone shots in each knee. While playing tennis recently, my patient heard a pop and ruptured his patellar tendon. I had to surgically repair it.                                   —ROBERT KLAPPER, M.D.

---

A tendon rupture is more serious since it nearly always requires surgery. Any tendon near the knee can tear, but ruptures of the quadriceps tendon and the patellar tendon are the two that will seriously incapacitate you. If the quad tendon is pulled away from its attachment at the 12 o'clock position of the kneecap, it leaves a palpable defect—a divot in the muscle and an inability to straighten the leg. (The quad tendon ruptures only in this one location.) The patellar tendon can rupture from either its attachment on the kneecap or its attachment on the tibia. Ruptures at the 6 o'clock position of the kneecap usually occur in sports-related injuries while ruptures at the tibial tubercle generally happen to people who have had previous knee surgery.

Irregardless of the location of the tendon rupture, the surgical treatment is the same. We make drill holes in the kneecap, put some stitches into the tendon, then thread the stitches through the kneecap. We tie the tendon back onto the bone and roughen up the bone a little so it will bleed and create a healing cascade that leads to scar formation.

If you've torn either your quad or patellar tendon, expect to be in a cast for six weeks. You'll have to face strenuous physical therapy once the cast is removed, but eventually you'll be as good as new.

## Patella Problems

Knee pain often originates in the patellofemoral joint, the place where the kneecap glides through the groove in the femur (the trochlea). Figures 3-5A and 3-5B are called the "sunrise" view

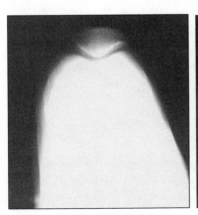 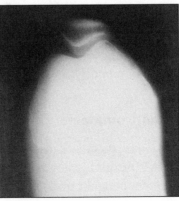

**3-5A (far left)**
This X ray of a knee is called the "sunrise" view. It shows the patella in its normal position, centered in its groove in the femur called the trochlea.

**3-5B (left)**
This sunrise view of the knee shows a patella that tracks badly, off to the side of the trochlea. This bad alignment leads to chondromalacia.

of the knee. Notice how the first X ray shows a patella tracking correctly, while the second X ray shows a patella tracking off to the side. (If the kneecap tracks badly, it is **always** laterally, off to the side, never medially, to the inside.) Hyaline cartilage coats both the surface of the trochlea and the back of the patella. If your patella doesn't slide smoothly in its groove, but tracks even slightly off-kilter, the result is increased wear on the cartilage (chondromalacia) in just the area where the excessive friction is occurring. The rest of the cartilage is left virtually unused.

To understand what's happening, look at the heels of your shoes. You have probably worn down a corner of the heel because of the way you walk. But if you had walked evenly on the heel, you would have equally distributed the wear over its entire surface. This same principle applies to the cartilage behind your kneecap: if you equally distribute the wear over the entire surface, you won't create uneven worn-out areas of cartilage. By strengthening the vastus medialis obliqus (VMO), the inner portion of your quadriceps muscles, to hold the kneecap in its proper position, you can force your kneecap to track more correctly and thereby distribute the load on the cartilage so that it lasts longer. Exercises in Chapter 10 and 11 help strengthen the VMO.

More women than men experience tracking problems, possibly because more women than men are knock-kneed. People with tracking problems usually have pain when going up and down stairs, walking or running downhill, or even sitting for long periods of time. This patellofemoral pain is one of the most troublesome areas of orthopedics.

## Chondromalacia

*Chondro* means cartilage and *malacia* means badness. Softening and cracking of the hyaline cartilage is called chondromalacia in its early stages. Most patients who first hear this diagnosis are under thirty, whereas patients over thirty will most likely have progressed to a later stage of cartilage damage called osteoarthritis (see below.)

Chondromalacia is classified from Grade 1 to Grade 4. Grade 1 is a softening or blistering of the cartilage, usually on the back of the patella. Grades 2 and 3 represent progressive steps in the worsening of the cracks and fissures in the cartilage. In Grade 4, the subchondral bone beneath the cartilage is exposed. Chondromalacia can be caused by a tracking problem as previously mentioned, or it can be simple genetics—at a certain age, your genetic clock turns on and the deterioration begins.

Surgery usually isn't recommended for this diagnosis because we're not very good at solving this problem surgically. Physical therapy is better for chondromalacia. The key is to strengthen the VMO, so that it can pull the vector of the kneecap toward the center and no longer let it track laterally (off to the side). You'll learn VMO strengthening exercises in Chapters 10 and 11.

---

**CHO-PAT KNEE STRAP**

A Cho-Pat Knee Strap can be placed around your knee to apply pressure to the patellar tendon thus guiding the kneecap in its groove. This improves tracking and spreads pressure more uniformly over the surface area. The Cho-Pat is waterproof, so you can wear it while participating in all water activities. Wear it only when you're active, not at rest.

---

## Osteoarthritis

Known as the "wear-and-tear" form of arthritis, osteoarthritis was formerly thought to be caused by excessive stress to the joints from high-impact activities. But more recent studies have shown that regular exercise does not predispose people to osteoarthritis. In fact, regular exercise can increase the functional capability of osteoarthritis patients.

Called OA for short, osteoarthritis usually strikes the weightbearing joints after the age of forty. We don't yet know the exact cause of OA, but obesity and family history are known to be risk factors. As we age, OA dries out the hyaline cartilage, deteriorating this protective cushion between the bones. This miraculous cartilage that provides such elegance to the joints is like your permanent teeth: you only get one set, so it is crucial to protect it. As OA progresses, the cartilage begins to grow brittle and to crack. Its surface may become pitted and uneven. There may even be "potholes" on the surface. Although OA begins in the hyaline cartilage and is primarily focused on the cartilage, it also affects other areas in and around the knee joint, including the muscles and tendons surrounding the joint and the subchondral bone at the ends of the bones just below the cartilage.

---

**SYMPTOMS OF ARTHRITIS**

The classic early symptom of arthritis is that you know when it's going to rain. When the barometer pressure is changing rapidly, you start to feel the deep, deep pain of arthritis. Other signs of arthritis specifically in the knee include swelling, pain, decreased range of motion and deformity. You may notice that you're becoming more bowlegged or more knock-kneed. If you have a high pain tolerance, you may not notice if you've begun to limp, but a friend or spouse may tell you.

---

Recently, the first state-by-state survey of arthritis in the United States showed that this condition is more common than previously thought. Instead of the forty million Americans believed to have arthritis, a Centers for Disease Control and Prevention survey showed that one in three Americans (seventy million people) suffers from some form of degenerative joint disease, primarily osteoarthritis.

## Posttraumatic Arthritis

Posttraumatic osteoarthritis is virtually the same thing as osteoarthritis except that it is caused by previous structural damage. The damage doesn't have to be in the knee, either. Trauma to any weightbearing joint—the lower back, the hip, knee, ankle, or foot—can cause eventual damage to adjacent joints. In fact, the injury doesn't even have to be on the same leg. A right ankle injury could cause problems with a left knee. **If you fractured your leg or your ankle years ago, the injury may have altered your gait so that you created stresses in your knee, leading to its early degeneration.**

Let's say you broke your knee as a child or a teenager. Doctors fixed it, but let's look at how it was "fixed." Picture yourself holding two plates. Imagine throwing one of them onto a concrete floor and seeing it smash into pieces. Even if you used the best glue possible and managed to put the jigsaw puzzle of pieces back together to form the perfect shape of the other plate, you would still see dozens of seams. Surgeons may have put your knee back together with plates and screws and whatever else it took to reconstruct the normal anatomy, but your body knows the difference. Years later, these irregularities begin to behave like fine sandpaper and, in the long run, they are enough to wear out the joint.

The symptoms for posttraumatic osteoarthritis are nearly the same as basic osteoarthritis. The only significant difference is that if surgery has taken place, pain could be coming from the hardware—the plates and screws that were used to reconstruct the tibia, femur, or patella. The tip of a piece of metal could be sticking into a muscle or other soft tissues, causing inflammation. In that case, removing the hardware could relieve your pain.

Posttraumatic arthritis is probably the easiest of all the categories of knee problems to diagnose, unless of course you've forgotten about childhood or adolescent injuries that could be the cause of today's orthopedic problems. When you carefully complete the body history questionnaire in Chapter 5, you may find clues regarding your current knee condition.

## Bursitis

There's only one bursa of importance in the knee: the pre-patellar bursa, which is located in front of the knee cap. When a carpenter or carpet layer works all day on his knees, he constantly applies pressure onto his knee caps, forcing them to work overtime. After a while, the viscosity of fluid inside the bursa sac changes, leading to bleeding and inflammation. Ice and rest are excellent treatments for bursitis, but it's even better not to aggravate the bursa in the first place. Don't kneel directly on your knees and don't squat as often. If you like to do activities close to the ground such as gardening, bring out a little stool or short chair to avoid squatting or kneeling.

## Cysts

A meniscal cyst can appear underneath the skin on either the medial (inside) or lateral (outside) side of the knee. In the early stages, these cysts may show up only on an MRI, but later they will create a visible ballooning along the joint line. By definition, this cyst is caused by a horizontal cleavage tear in the meniscus (see illustration 3-2, Part A on page 40) that behaves like a one-way valve, allowing joint fluid from the inside of your knee to leak out behind the meniscus and collect just beneath the skin. Repairing this meniscus tear is a bad idea; it will fail. The correct treatment for a meniscal cyst is to trim away arthroscopically the horizontal tear in the meniscus, eliminating the one-way valve so that the cyst can drain back into the joint and resolve itself. The worst thing you can do is remove the cyst from the outside and not do the arthroscopic procedure. If you don't get to the root cause, which is the meniscal tear, the cyst will keep coming back.

A Baker cyst, located behind the knee, is caused by a thinness at the back of the knee joint capsule that allows fluid to collect there. Nearly fifteen percent of all people have this anatomical deformity in the knee, but most people can live happily ever after with it, since it rarely causes pain or loss of function. However, if you've had a Baker's cyst for years and now you're noticing increased swelling and discomfort, something new may have happened inside your knee. Perhaps early arthritic changes are occurring, or maybe you've torn a meniscus, both of which can cause an increase of fluid in the joint. That fluid will try to escape wherever it can, so it goes into the Baker cyst. This means that the cyst isn't the real problem; it's only a symptom of some other condition. The cyst will go down once you take care of what's causing the inflammation in your knee. Surgery to remove the Baker cyst should be avoided, because the cyst will simply grow back. Consider an inflamed Baker cyst a signal that you need an **MRI** (see page 122) to see if you tore your meniscus or to see if anything else has degenerated.

## Fractures and Stress Fractures

A fracture is a break in a bone and is usually caused by trauma such as a fall or an accident. If the pieces are pulled apart, the fracture is considered displaced; if the pieces are not pulled apart, it is considered non-displaced. A stress fracture is a break in a bone so subtle that it won't show up on an X ray; it takes a bone scan or an MRI to view a stress fracture. Any of these fractures may cause you pain, swelling, bruising, tenderness, or an inability to move your knee.

If your fracture or stress fracture is near the knee, you and your doctor need to be aggressive in keeping you immobilized and non-weightbearing. You need to be on crutches and restrict movement for six weeks. You don't have to be in a cast; a knee immobilizer or brace may be all that's needed to keep you from using your knee. You can remove the immobilizer at night to bend and straighten your knee gently, which squeezes joint fluid into and out of the joint for nourishment. If you don't take these measures, you could move the pieces of bone apart, turning a nondisplaced fracture into a displaced one, which would mean you'd need surgery to put the two pieces of bone back together correctly. (Fractures that remain nondisplaced generally won't need surgery.) Granted, without moving for six weeks, your muscles and tendons will atrophy, your knee will be stiff, and, afterward, you'll have to work hard in physical therapy to regain your strength and range of motion. But this is necessary, because the number one priority is to get the bone to heal correctly. Afterward, you can address the health of the soft tissues surrounding the knee.

With **any** kind of fracture near the knee, a major concern is whether the path of the break runs into the joint, thereby interrupting the cartilage. If the surface of the cartilage is disrupted, if there's any incongruity that violates the smooth cartilage surfaces on the end of the femur, on the top of the tibia, or behind the patella, you'll end up with an irregularity that years later will behave like sand paper and create posttraumatic osteoarthritis. (See page 53.)

The most common fracture of the knee is of the tibial plateau, the top of the shin bone where the hyaline cartilage covers the bone. Picture a golf tee: it's shaped similarly to your tibia, with a flat surface on top and a long shaft. Imagine the golf tee being split in half so the top of the tee is cracked. The way to put it back together is to squeeze the two pieces together, and if the wooden tee were made of cartilage on top and subchondral bone below, it would heal itself by mending the break both in the cartilage and the bone. However, no matter how perfectly the two pieces of the cartilage are put together, there will always be a seam, and that seam can later cause post-traumatic OA.

If the fracture in your tibial plateau isn't a simple split but is accompanied by a depression in the bone, the surgeon will have to drill a hole and punch the depressed portion of that bone back into place. Then, to ensure that the bone stays where it belongs, a bone graft must be placed underneath to keep it from collapsing.

A "chip" fracture of your knee is actually a ligament injury. If the ligament is torn off the bone and pulls a piece of the bony anchoring site with it, that's called a chip or an avulsion fracture, but it will be treated like a ligament sprain. Some consider it advantageous to have the ligament interrupted at the bone rather than in its fleshy portion, because once the bone reattaches, the original ligament length is maintained. I, however, the fleshy portion of the ligament is disrupted, it can potentially heal longer than normal, leaving a knee that feels loose and has decreased stability.

If you shattered your knee cap, think twice before allowing your doctor to put the pieces back together. Trying to piece together a patella with pins and wires is a no-win situation. Here's what I do instead: I remove the tiny pieces of the shattered knee cap. I keep the biggest piece I can find, smooth down the rough edges, and reattach the tendon and the muscle to that one piece. This essentially gives the patient a mini-knee cap that's in one piece, so it doesn't need wires or pins. It won't fall apart, there aren't any wires to break, and there won't be any irregular pieces scratching away the trochlea to cause posttraumatic arthritis in the future.

---

**SHATTERED KNEE CAP?**
Ask your surgeon about having a partial patellectomy. By removing all the small, shattered pieces of the patella and keeping just the largest piece, you'll have better range of motion, you won't need a second surgery to remove the hardware, and you won't be creating future arthritis.

---

## Spurs, Contractures, and Adhesions

As the hyaline cartilage in your knee breaks down with age, the joint space narrows and the bones are no longer at their usual distance from each other. The body senses that change in distance and thinks there's laxity or looseness in the joint, so it lays down bone in the form of spurs to try to stabilize the knee again. While spurs do make the knee more stable, they also act like speed bumps in a parking lot—they slow down the knee's movement. They also cause pain, swelling, and reduced motion.

A muscle or capsule contracture is a persistent constriction of those tissues, which causes pain and limitation of movement. The most common contracture of the knee is a flexion contracture in which the knee remains slightly bent at all times. People with flexion contractures make themselves comfortable by putting a pillow under their bent knees, by walking less, and by sitting in their lounge chairs more. By catering to this limitation, they begin falling into the Negative Spiral shown on page 37.

Adhesions are scar tissue formed by the body following inflammation, injury, or surgery. You need enough scar tissue for healing to take place, but you don't want an overabundance of scar tissue, because that creates it own problems of limited motion and pain. Think of adhesions in this way: tissues that should normally be separate and move independently are now adhered (stuck) together. You lose your normal, smooth flow of motion; you feel muscles or joints tugging on each other as you move.

Scar tissue and normal tissue look very different under a microscope. Normal tissue appears well-organized, like a beautifully-woven rug, while scar tissue looks very disorganized: picture a hundred fish nets tossed randomly on top of each other with the strands of the nets going in different directions. What had been separate, lubricated planes of skin, connective tissue, subcutaneous fat, blood vessels, nerves, and muscles have become a compacted, rubbery mass of scar tissue that is thicker and harder, and therefore less elastic, than normal tissues. The irregular nature of scar tissue blocks free circulation and limits drainage of the blood vessels and other fluids through the lymphatic system, because there's no organized anatomy, no specific blood or lymph vessels to take fluid away through the mass of scar tissue. Thus what often accompanies scar tissue is stiffness, swelling, and pain. Yet immature scar tissue—a weak, stiff, nonlubricated mass of disorganized fibers—eventually evolves into mature, normalized tissues that are strong, pliable, and well-organized. Your body creates a scar that functions normally again.

In spite of the various things that can go wrong with your knees, there are steps you can take to alleviate the pain, instability, and limited function that accompany these conditions. You can immediately begin the self-treatments suggested in Chapter 7 and start the pool and land exercise programs presented in Chapters 10 and 11. But first, you'll learn how to modify your exercise routine to stop hurting your knees in Chapter 4.

# 4 STOP HURTING YOUR KNEES

Many people with sore knees have never exercised. Others haven't exercised in years or have exercised far too little. But a large number have damaged their weightbearing joints, especially their knees, by playing abusive sports with a passion. There is a growing epidemic of knee problems, especially in aging baby boomers who are devoted to running, skiing, tennis, basketball, volleyball, or racquetball, and who, because they aren't built for these sports or haven't had coaching to learn proper body mechanics, have created knee problems with every workout, race, or game.

Yet they continue to pursue abusive activities with excessive regularity.

A safe guess would be that only ten to twenty percent of the population is anatomically built to run, yet we see people by the hundreds awkwardly slogging their way through miles and miles of workouts and races with their knees splayed asymmetrically and their hands and feet flailing. Such clumsy runners are creating knee problems with every step! We have many of them as patients. We also see tennis players with knees sore from playing three sets every day and body builders who follow weight-training programs with no rest or variety programmed into their weekly schedules. These patients tell us they can barely stand up without pain after sitting in a car or going to a movie.

You, too, may be participating in a physical activity that is absolutely wrong for your knee anatomy. You may be focusing on a single sport and doing too much of it, causing overuse injuries. You may be using a stair-climbing machine or attending step classes, both highly abusive to knees even in small doses. Leg-press machines and treadmills are other culprits, as are aerobic classes. If your knees hurt, these may be the cause of your pain.

---

**A WAKE-UP CALL**

If knee pain has interrupted your daily workouts, consider it a wake-up call. Use this time to learn to read your body's monitoring systems and learn to interpret the messages your body sends you with its pain signals. Always move away from activities that increase pain and gravitate toward those that do not.

---

To visualize how injuries occur from abuse and overuse, pinch the skin on the back of your hand, then let the skin go and watch what happens. You'll see the skin **slowly** settling and flattening—slowly, because as you age the elasticity in all your tissues decays. Your skin, muscles, ligaments, tendons, and joints don't bounce back instantly the way they did when you were ten years old.

This lack of elasticity means that you shouldn't repetitively bang on your muscles, ligaments, tendons, or knee joints without being alert to potential damage. Think of how you tear an old credit card in two: either you cut it in half with scissors or you fold it back and forth, back and forth until eventually you make a white fatigue line. And then the card easily tears in half. Or it snaps. That's exactly what you're doing to your body with repetitive-strain injuries. Running too many miles, playing too much tennis, lifting too many pounds, or skiing too many moguls **when your knees are warning you to stop** is a sure way to create an increasingly serious knee problem.

**Your knees are your responsibility and you must assume all risk for them.** By selecting your physical activities more wisely, you can have an injury-free sport or fitness program.

Exercise comes in two flavors: nurturing and abusive. The sports people love most—the sports previously mentioned—abuse the body's weightbearing joints, especially the knees, whereas pool exercise, bicycling, and working out on ski machines such as the Nordic Track remove impact from the weightbearing joints and are therefore nurturing. Most people don't consider the abusiveness of their exercise routines until pain or physical limitation strikes. At that point, they pay attention.

If you're reading this chapter, **you're probably ready to consider changing the flavor of your exercise program.** Our hope is that you'll begin nurturing exercise on a regular basis. By using safe forms of exercise **most of the time** to maintain and enhance fitness, you may be able to continue **occasionally** your beloved sports and activities for many years to come.

In this chapter we can help you:

- Find and include a variety of nurturing activities in your exercise routines
- Make a successful transition to your new nurturing activity
- Set sensible training limits
- Identify injuries in the making and prevent them by paying attention to early warning signs
- Resolve to take rest days
- Use ice, heat, and other self-treatments to reduce pain, stiffness, and swelling from overuse injuries
- Manage your knee injury and speed your recovery

- Learn anatomical predispositions to knee injuries and identify activities to avoid if you have such predispositions
- Do self treatments for immediate pain relief.
- Understand the need for lifelong management of your knee condition

## NURTURING ACTIVITIES

The nurturing exercises we suggest, in this order of preference, are pool workouts, bicycling, and the use of a ski machine. Your task here and throughout this chapter is to discover what movements **your body** responds to without discomfort. You may love bicycling, which for most people is a smooth, nurturing exercise, but for you the biking movement might cause pain in your back or hips. Or you may love working out on a ski machine, but a back injury keeps you from maintaining the balance required. Perhaps you love gliding effortlessly through water, but find that a pool's chlorine irritates your skin. Try all three programs. Factor in your body's reactions to each and choose at least one of these three nurturing exercises that can help you stop hurting your knees. If you can do all three, the optimum crosstraining program to prevent future knee problems is to rotate between them.

### Pool Program

A pool program is our first choice for a nurturing workout because exercising in water offers many bonuses. These include:

BALANCED STRENGTH IN MUSCLE PAIRS. Back and forth movements of the arms, legs, and trunk are possible only because muscles work in synchronized pairs—when one contracts, the opposing one relaxes. Although you could forget to strengthen one half of a muscle pair on land, that can't happen in water. Every exercise in water forces you to work both halves of each muscle pair. For every push forward against water's resistance, you must pull backward to the starting position. For every swing upward, you must swing downward. When you exercise in water, symmetry is built in.

**AEROBIC AND ANAEROBIC FITNESS.** Aerobic fitness allows for moderate, continuous endurance exercise such as hiking for six miles without stopping. Anaerobic fitness is necessary for strenuous bursts of speed and explosive power, such as running up a flight of stairs. Both aerobic and anaerobic fitness are vital to a well-conditioned person. If you suffer from knee pain, it may be impossible for you even to think of performing such activities on land. In water, however, sore knees are often capable of walking, running, and even jumping, so that aerobic work is achieved effortlessly and anaerobic work sneaks in almost painlessly. You can feel a sense of improved strength against the water's resistance, yet because of the greatly-reduced gravitational pull, you should encounter little pain in the workout and end it feeling fresh.

**IMPROVED FLEXIBILITY.** Although stretching on land is a peaceful and soothing activity for most people, for knee patients it can produce discomfort and strain. In water you'll find that you can assume positions to perform stretches that you couldn't possibly perform on land.

**IMPROVED BALANCE.** In water you are constantly using your abdominal and back muscles as well as your arms and legs to maintain erect body alignment and balance. Increased strength in these muscles, plus focus on a constantly-changing balance point in water, will lead to improved balance on land that will carry over into your daily activities. Further, improved flexibility and balance are equally important in preventing falls.

**Increased range of motion**. The water's buoyancy offers you a somewhat unexpected gift. You'll find that your knee can bend and straighten, that you can squat and rise more easily than you ever would be able to on land. Water's buoyancy will naturally allow you increased mobility each session without your having to think about it.

**Increased coordination.** When you walk or run on land, your right arm and left leg move at the same time: this is called cross-crawl patterning. In water, many people become disoriented regarding the opposition of their limbs. It may take some practice and attention to master this, but the result will be worth the effort, for water training increases overall coordination by virtue of its emphasis on cross-crawl patterning, which is the basis of all human coordination.

**Improved gait.** Because of ongoing knee pain, you may have developed an uneven walking pattern or gait and you may have lost strength in the quadriceps or hamstring muscles. The gait training in Exercises 12 and 13 on pages 173 to 175 will help you create new habit patterns that are symmetrical and balanced at the same time as they force new strength into the weak muscles.

**A sense of well-being.** What an amazing change in attitude you can experience as soon as you enter the water! Stress washes away. You'll stop working on your problems, take a deep breath, and notice that your shoulders and neck have relaxed. You'll feel better simply for having submerged in water. You'll find a full, satisfying pool workout in Chapter 10.

## Bicycle Program

Bicycling nurtures your weightbearing joints (back, hips, knees, feet, and lower legs) because you don't have the full weight of your body crashing into those joints as you ride. Additionally, the cycling motion uses the hinge joint part of the knee's function only; it doesn't place any rotational torque on the knee. The menisci and cruciate ligaments inside the knee joint are particularly susceptible to injury due to rotational movements, so by eliminating rotation, such as the twisting of racquetball or the pivoting of basketball, the source of many knee injuries is also eliminated. Further, biking focuses primarily on the **quadriceps muscles, the source of key protection for the knees.**

Athletes and former athletes generally prefer the traditional bike on which you sit upright. Older people and those with back problems often prefer the recumbent bike, which lets you sit closer to the ground with your legs pumping in front of you. Most gyms have both bikes, so give each a solid try. Ride one to see how you feel, followed the next day by a ride on the other to test its effects. Let your body tell you which bike feels better. Then, should you buy a bike for your home you'll have a preference based on experience rather than on the word of a salesperson. Both bikes have straps on the pedals, which let you use the quads and hamstrings to maintain balanced strength in both halves of the quads/hamstrings muscle pair. Without straps you would strictly use the quads to push down on the pedals, but with straps you can pull up with one leg while pushing down with the other.

Former athletes often need the thrill of the open road or bike path plus the rush of the wind in their faces to satisfy their athletic appetites, but if those qualities aren't absolutely necessary to you, use an indoor stationary bike, which provides an uninterrupted ride, thus a smoother workout for your muscles and joints. Stopping and going at traffic lights, for instance, breaks up the blood flow and lubrication of the joints. It's wiser to work your tissues gradually and consistently, rather then reacting to traffic and the environment with sudden stops and starts.

Think of an old rubber band. If you pull on it slowly at first and gradually warm it up, you can get it to do its job.

But if you suddenly pull it wide open, it may break. Your tendons, muscles, ligaments, and other tissues react the same way. They appreciate a **gentle, consistent warm-up** and a steady workout. If you go outdoors, choose a location with the fewest traffic lights and other interruptions to a steady ride. Use easy gears so pushing the pedals is comfortable. **Don't push hard gears that can strain the knees**.

---

**MOUNTAIN BIKES**

Although mountain biking generally allows for an uninterrupted ride, it presents potential dangers. Weigh the soul satisfaction you'll receive against the possible risks before you begin peddling. Consider your fitness level, the elevation gains and losses, the condition of the trail (narrow? rocky? slippery? sandy?), then judge whether you and your knees are up to the challenge.

---

### *Stationary Bike Program*

Perhaps the most important part of your biking program is setting the height of your seat. Ideally the person who sets it should be a knowledgeable bike rider. If you must set it for yourself, start by making sure the seat is flat, not tilted up or down at the front. An improper angle on the seat can cause deep soreness in the crotch. Next, sit comfortably and place your feet under the straps. The balls of your feet, not your arches, should be centered over the pedals, and both feet should remain flat through the entire range of motion in order to push the maximum force through the pedals.

Keep one foot flat, not pointed toward the ground, and push that foot down to its lowest point in the circle. Set your seat so you can maintain a twenty-degree bend in your knees as each foot passes through this lowest position. That's the key to setting your seat correctly. If your knee straightens fully instead of retaining the twenty-degree bend, your seat is too high and should be lowered. If your knees bend more than twenty degrees at that lowest point, you could create patellofemoral pain (behind the kneecap) or hip pain. Raise the seat to a higher position.

Good biking form dictates that you keep your knees and feet pointed straight ahead. Bad form can create knee, hip, and ankle pain. Keep your arms relaxed and bent at the elbows. If you ride with your arms straight and tense, the muscular tension in the arms is transferred into your shoulders and neck.

Set the bike's control for no resistance and start peddling slowly as you warm up. Stop if you feel sharp pain. Slow if a mild ache increases in intensity; you may have started peddling too quickly. You can often work through soreness and pain if you **gradually** increase speed, then gradually slow, then increase your speed again. On your first bike workout, let the first five minutes be a warm up in which you constantly evaluate what your knees are feeling. Adjust your speed accordingly. During this time of restructuring your fitness regimen, you want to learn when to slow, when to stop, and when you can work through pain.

If biking doesn't increase your knee pain during the warm-up, continue on for fourteen minutes the first day (low resistance, low revolutions). If your knees aren't sore the next day, add two minutes at your next workout for a sixteen-minute ride. Add two minutes each workout until you reach thirty minutes. After you perform a pain-free, thirty-minute bike ride, **then** you can start increasing the resistance, **but not before**. This resistance is equivalent to the stack of weights in a weight room, and, as you know, you can injure yourself by trying to lift too much too soon.

Most stationary bikes have ten to twelve levels of resistance that can be changed at the touch of a button. You started at 0 resistance the first day. Now, after your thirty-minute, pain-free ride, you're ready to move to Level 1. Return again to a fourteen-minute ride the first day. Add two minutes every workout until you reach thirty minutes at Level 1. Now, assuming you're still pain-free, you're ready to move to Level 2 to start again at fourteen minutes. **(If you have a flare-up of knee pain, you must cut back the resistance until you've returned to a pain-free state during biking.)** When you work your way up to twenty-four minutes at Level 2, try riding the first fourteen minutes at Level 2 and the last ten minutes at Level 3. Once you improve your knee strength and fitness, try some interesting variations, such as placing your bike in front of the TV and riding for the first quarter of a basketball game: sprint during fast breaks and ride more slowly as shots are set up and rebounds taken. Eventually, over a few months, you may be able to ride through an entire game. Not a sports fan? Watch your favorite half-hour sitcom, sprinting through the commercials and riding more slowly during the dialogue.

Here's a more athletic variation: ride at Level 1 for one minute, Level 2 for two minutes, Level 3 for three minutes, and so on up to Level 5, then work your way back down with four minutes at Level 4, three minutes at Level 3, until you're back at Level 1. If biking agrees with you and you claim it as your primary nurturing exercise, you'll want to buy some stiff-shank biking shoes, which, by design, harness all of your muscular force and transmit it through the pedals for maximum performance.

---

### USE OF A BIKE STAND

If you wish to ride your own road or mountain bike in a safer, indoor environment during foul weather, buy a bike stand. Remove the bike's front wheel and let the back wheel spin over the stand's roller. Assume your familiar position on the bike and play with the gears instead of hitting buttons to change levels on a regular stationary bike.

## Ski Machines

Ski machines offer low-impact, weightbearing exercise, which is nurturing because you are not picking up and forcing down your feet. There's no jarring of the hips, back, or knees. And here's a bonus to skiing: the machine helps you develop agility, coordination, and balance while you maintain your aerobic fitness. Ski machines strengthen your mid-body, because those muscles are constantly working to stabilize you in an upright stance. Your neck is constantly working, too, so **if your neck is weak, stiff, sore, or injured, choose one of the other nurturing exercises or start very slowly and progress extremely gradually.**

There are two types of ski machines—dependent and independent. Dependent models link the motion of the skis: when you move one ski forward, the other ski moves backward automatically. Skiing on independent models is a harder skill to master, but offers more authentic skiing simulation and a more vigorous workout. Try out both of these machines more than once at the store because they can be frustrating at first and require several attempts before you'll feel comfortable enough to make a choice. Consider the cumbersome size of these machines. If your space is small, look for a ski machine that collapses to be placed under a high bed or against a wall.

Start by learning the basic stance and balance on the machine. Step into the footholds, grasp the security handles, and begin moving your legs in the forward-gliding motion used in cross-country skiing. Then let go of the security handles and grasp the machine's hand pulleys. Swing your arms and legs in opposition to each other: right arm forward with left leg then left arm forward with right leg. Keep trying until the movements become smooth. Don't get frustrated—it may take a few sessions or even a few weeks to feel comfortable, just as it does with real skiing.

While some fitness experts say that badly-aligned knees don't belong on a ski machine, since straight alignment is forced upon them, others believe that being bowlegged or knock-kneed is not an issue. You'll have to consider yourself a test case of one and give it a try.

### Ski Machine Program

Experiment with your new ski machine three or four times in the first week, becoming accustomed to the way it moves and how your body feels while using it. If you're uncertain as to whether your knee condition can tolerate the use of a ski machine, try it for a brief four minutes the first day, Day 1. Evaluate how your knee feels the next day, Day 2. If you don't have increased knee pain or discomfort, ski for six minutes on Day 3. Evaluate again on Day 4; and if you feel fine, ski for eight minutes on Day 5. Follow this pattern of adding two minutes every-other day until you reach twenty minutes. If you've felt confident on a ski machine in the past, start with eight minutes and add two minutes every-other day until you reach twenty minutes.

**Anyone over 50 who isn't fit should start with four minutes on Day 1 and increase skiing time by just one minute every-other day.**

Regardless of whether you're uncertain or confident, fit or unfit, ski at a rate that you perceive to be "easy" until you've worked your way up to twenty minutes. If your muscles are sore or if you feel tired at this stage of your build-up, continue with the twenty-minute sessions for two weeks, skiing every-other day. Once you work through the soreness and fatigue, you can begin another build-up: add two minutes to your every-other-day skiing program until you reach thirty minutes. Continue the 30-minute skiing sessions until they no longer seem challenging and you no longer experience soreness or fatigue.

The next step is to increase your speed until you perceive an exertion level of "moderate," while reducing the duration of your workout to twenty minutes. Add two minutes at each moderate-level workout (scheduled every other day) until you work your way back up to thirty minutes. This may feel like a slow and guarded approach, but slow progression minimizes injury and maximizes your safety and enjoyment.

After a month of moderate, thirty-minute workouts, attempt a "hard" workout, one in which you breathe heavily and feel fatigue both during and after the workout. Evaluate how you feel the next day. If you have no flare-up of knee pain, do one hard workout a week mixed in with your moderate ones. For variety, you can try interval training: a work period is followed by a recovery period, followed by another work period, and so on. Try one minute of easy skiing, two minutes of moderate skiing, one minute of slow recovery, then one minute of hard skiing. Repeat, moving slowly through the first  minute of recovery before beginning the next work period. You can create your own intervals measured either by the clock or TV. Ski hard during commercials or action sequences, then slower during the talking.

Another variation you can try is to alternate between short strides, which tax your thigh muscles, and long strides, which make you work the muscles in your buttocks. Do two minutes of short strides followed by two minutes of long strides, then recover slowly for two minutes. Repeat.

## SUCCESSFUL TRANSITION TO YOUR NURTURING ACTIVITY

You've grown to love certain sports and activities throughout your lifetime because those activities give you the most satisfaction and pleasure—even joy. You've worked hard to master the details of your game or fitness routine, and it won't be easy to walk away from that integral part of your life. Acknowledge that there will be a transition time until your body and mind adapt to the new movements. Perhaps a lifetime of successful tennis became part of your identity —it may take weeks before you **will** feel the same pride in your bicycling prowess. Or if you loved crossing the finish line at road races, it might be a while before you sense the same pleasure of pushing deeply past your fitness level, "going beyond" the pain into a new accomplishment of speed—but you **can** do just that in your pool workouts. Maybe the step aerobics class at your gym was the most fun you'd had in years, but you **will** find rhythmic, swinging pleasure using a ski machine once you master it.

Like anything new, it takes time for your mind to become part of the activity. It takes a while before your body begins performing the skills automatically, as if taking **you** for a ride. Remind yourself that you're making a life-long change in your fitness routine in order to heal your knees. Give yourself whatever time that change will take.

---

### DO SIX WORKOUTS BEFORE EVALUATING

Over-achievers often get frustrated when they don't see immediate progress. When I work with elite athletes who are making a "come-back" after injury, I always tell them "Just put your head down and do six workouts. Don't look up until we've finished them. Then we'll see how you're doing." Apply this same logic to your transition from abusive to nurturing sports. Do six workouts without judging anything. Then you'll have gained enough fitness and skill to evaluate your progress in making this new activity your own.          —LYNDA HUEY

# Huey-Klapper Knee-Point Assessment

Circle numbers in each column that describe your current condition.
Total each column in boxes A & B (be sure to include 100 base points).

| | Base Points | Deductions |
|---|---|---|
| Start wiith 100 points | (100) | |
| Under 30 | 30 | |
| Under 40 | 20 | |
| Age 45-55 | | 10 |
| Over 55 | | 20 |
| Over 65 | | 30 |
| Good form during exercise | 10 | |
| No training on good form | | 10 |
| History of knee problems (but not currently) | | 10 |
| Current knee problems (no surgery) | | 20 |
| Ideal body weight | 10 | |
| Overweight 20 lbs. | | 10 |
| Overweight 30 lbs. | | 20 |
| Overweight 40 lbs. or more | | 30 |
| Slightly knock-kneed or bowlegged | | 10 |
| Badly-aligned knees | | 30 |
| Knee pain after exercise | | 10 |
| Knee instability | | 20 |
| Knee surgery (over 1 year ago, after age 18) | | 30 |
| Knee surgery less than 9 months ago | | 40 |
| Knee surgery less than 6 months ago | | 50 |
| Knee surgery less than 3 months ago | | 60 |

**Total each column as it applies to you:**   A [ ]      B [ ]

Total Base Points (write number from box A here:)   [ ] A

Total Deductions (write number from box B here:)   − [ ] B

**Subtract box B from box A**   = [ ]

*This is your recommended total Knee Points per week.*

# The Huey-Klapper Knee-Point Scale

All point values shown are for **one hour** of that activity. For longer or shorter periods, modify points accordingly (divide in half for thirty minutes of activity, etc.)

| Activity | Points | Activity | Points |
|---|---|---|---|
| Aerobics class | 9 | Run – grass, dirt, track | 12 |
| Aerobics class – low impact | 6 | Run – striding on track | 12 |
| Ballet class – barre work | 6 | Ski machine | 0 |
| Ballet class – floor work | 9 | Skiing – cross-country | 6 |
| Baseball | 6 | Skiing – downhill, bumps | 24 |
| Basketball | 24 | Skiing – downhill, groomed, no bumps | 12 |
| Bicycling – stationary | 0 | Soccer | 12 |
| Bicycling – road bike, flat | 0 | Softball | 12 |
| Bicycling – road bike, some hills | 6 | Stair-climbing machine | 12 |
| Bicycling – mountain bike | 12 | Step aerobics class | 12 |
| Body boarding – no fins | 0 | Stretching (non-weightbearing) | 0 |
| Body boarding – fins | 3 | Surfing (no knee paddling) | 3 |
| Elliptical training machine | 6 | Surfing (knee paddling) | 6 |
| Football – contact | 12 | Swimming – crawl | 0 |
| Football – touch/flag | 12 | Swimming – breast stroke | 18 |
| Golf – riding in cart | 0 | Tennis – doubles | 6 |
| Golf – walking | 6 | Tennis – singles | 12 |
| Hiking – mostly flat | 3 | Therapy exercises for knees | 0 |
| Hiking – some hills | 6 | Treadmill walking | 12 |
| Hiking – steep hills | 9 | Volleyball – beach | 12 |
| Kickboxing | 12 | Volleyball – indoors | 18 |
| Martial arts | 12 | Walking – flat | 6 |
| Pilates – mat | 0 | Walking – hills | 12 |
| Pilates – reformer | 12 | Weight training – total body | 12 |
| Pool workout | 0 | Weight training – lower body | 12 |
| Racquetball | 12 | Weight training – upper body | 0 |
| Rugby | 24 | Yoga – standing poses | 9 |
| Run – asphalt, concrete | 18 | Yoga – lying, sitting poses | 3 |

## TRAINING LIMITS

Depending on your sports background and training knowledge, you may be able to set your own training limits by planning a wise blend of nurturing activities along with an **occasional** soul-satisfying foray into your favorite but abusive sport. Most people, however, need guidance identifying **and limiting** the abusive exercises in their weekly routine.

The Huey-Klapper Knee-Point Scale on the facing page lists many popular sports and fitness activities. It will help you identify the sports you should increase in your healthy-knee lifestyle and the ones you should limit. Notice that each hour of workout is given a point value. The most nurturing activities are 0 points; the most abusive ones are 24 points. The other activities fall somewhere between.

Start a list to keep track of the points in your weekly workout routine. Write the day at the top of the page and list everything you did that day, whether it was planned exercise or unavoidable exercise such as walking fifteen minutes in a parking garage to find your car. Look at the Huey-Klapper Scale to assign a point value to your activities. Add or subtract more points depending on how long you continued. Keep this list going for one full week, then tally all your points for a grand weekly total.

Your point total may be as high as 130 to 190 points. If so, that's a clue to your current problem. **You've probably been hurting your knees with too much abusive activity.** So how many points are right for you? Your age, your weight, your knee alignment, your good or bad form while performing your activities, and your history of knee problems or surgeries will tell you how much you should limit your activities. Think of it this way: just as people count calories to control their weight, you can now count activity points to see if you're nurturing or abusing your knees. The chart on page 75 shows you how to determine your weekly recommended point total. Start with 100 points, then add and subtract points as they apply to your **current situation today.** The number you arrive at is your critical threshold for the week: **stay under that number to maintain optimal knee fitness.**

If you've exceeded your safe point limit, consider ways you can reduce your point total by running on grass, by walking instead of running, by playing doubles tennis instead of singles, and by substituting nurturing activities for two or more abusive-sports days. Notice that pool work-outs, swimming the crawl, and using stationary bikes and ski machines are 0 points. So is biking on flat terrain, stretching, and doing the therapy exercises that appear in Chapter 11. It may take a calculator plus an hour or two of creative thinking to plan a safe yet vigorous program that satisfies you. Don't fret. If you don't like your first stab at a new nurturing program, you can always change it the next week and the week after that until you're pleased with it. Try out as many low-point activities as you wish to make it easier to stay beneath your critical threshold.

Keep a weekly log of the points you spend in all your activities. After a month you should begin to see the pattern: the weeks with the low point totals are knee friendly. You'll start becoming frugal with your points, rationing them wisely over the week while at the same time saving your knees from continued abuse and damage.

Keep your goal firmly in mind: you want to be able to continue the sports you love on an occasional basis, so keep them that—strictly occasional—and do nurturing exercises for your daily fitness maintenance. This may sound like a huge sacrifice at first, but as soon as you realize you're saving your knees for years to come, you'll start savoring your once-a-week run, basketball game, or tennis match as pleasure enough into exchange for your knees.

Review the sample workouts that follow for ideas on how to change your abusive fitness routine into a more nurturing one for your knees.

## Tennis Sample

Rod is a tall, stocky, sixty-eight-year-old tennis player who plays with good form and no history of knee problems. He followed this program for years before his knees recently started bothering him:

| | | | |
|---|---|---|---|
| Monday | Tennis—3 sets of singles | 2 hours | **24 points** |
| Tuesday | Tennis—3 sets of doubles | 2 hours | **12 points** |
| Wednesday | Walking—hills | 90 minutes | **18 points** |
| Thursday | Tennis—3 sets of doubles | 2 hours | **12 points** |
| Friday | Tennis—3 sets of singles | 2 hours | **24 points** |
| Saturday | Swim—Breast stroke | 30 minutes | **9 points** |
| Sunday | Rest | | |
| | | **Total Points:** | **99** |

Using the chart on page 75, he gave himself 100 points, then added these points:

| | |
|---|---|
| Good form during exercise | 10 points |
| **Points to add in Box A:** | **10 points** |

Then he subtracted these points:

| | |
|---|---|
| Over 65 years of age | 30 points |
| Current knee problems | 20 points |
| Overweight 30 pounds | 20 points |
| Knee pain after exercise | <u>10 points</u> |
| **Points to subtract in Box B:** | **80 points** |

Thus his formula looks like this: **100 + 10 = 110 − 80 = 30 points.**

He decided to modify his sports life immediately; he dropped down to the 27 points per week shown in the box below. Notice that Rod added the stretching and land therapy exercises for knees shown in Chapter 11. He stopped doing the breast stroke and switched to the crawl. **(Breast stroke should be avoided by anyone with knee pain!)** He's doing a ski machine workout two days a week. And he continues to play tennis two days a week, sticking to doubles, which are kinder to knees than singles.

| | | | |
|---|---|---|---|
| Monday | Stretch | 15 minutes | **0 points** |
| | Tennis—3 sets of doubles | 90 minutes | **9 points** |
| Tuesday | Swim—crawl | 2 x 30 minutes | **0 points** |
| | Therapy exercises for knees | 30 minutes | **0 points** |
| Wednesday | Bicycling—road bike, hills | 90 minutes | **9 points** |
| | Stretch | 30 minutes | **0 point** |
| Thursday | Ski Machine | 30 minutes | **0 point** |
| | Therapy exercises for knees | 30 minutes | **0 points** |
| Friday | Stretch | 15 minutes | **0 points** |
| | Tennis—3 sets of doubles | 90 minutes | **9 points** |
| Saturday | Swim—crawl | 30 minutes | **0 points** |
| | Ski machine | 30 minutes | **0 point** |
| | Therapy exercises for knees | 30 minutes | **0 points** |
| Sunday | **Rest Day** | | |
| | | **Total Points:** | <u>27</u> |

## Running Sample

Julie is a forty-nine-year-old woman who loved to run long distances nearly every day and compete in 10K and half-marathon races on the week-ends. She came to running late so never received high school or college coaching. She is slightly knock-kneed, and her running form is suspect. This is what her weekly program looked like before severe knee pain hit during a race:

| | | | |
|---|---|---|---|
| Monday | Run 9 miles on roads | 1 hour | **18 points** |
| | Yoga class: 1/2 standing and 1/2 lying and sitting poses | 1 hour | **6 points** |
| Tuesday | Run 7 miles on grass | 45 minutes | **9 points** |
| | Weight training—total body | 30 minutes | **12 points** |
| Wednesday | Run sprints on track | 1 hour | **12 points** |
| | Pool workout | 30 minutes | **0 points** |
| Thursday | Run 12 miles on roads | 90 minutes | **27 points** |
| | Stretch | 15 minutes | **0 points** |
| Friday | Run 5 miles on roads | 35 minutes | **10 points** |
| | Yoga class: Lying and sitting poses | 1 hour | **3 points** |
| Saturday | Warm-up 2 miles | 16 minutes | **5 points** |
| | Stretch | 15 minutes | **0 points** |
| | Road race—half marathon | 90 minutes | **27 points** |
| Sunday | Pool workout—deep | 1 hour | **0 points** |
| | | **Total Points:** | **129** |

Julie realized she needed to improve her running form, so she found a good coach who has already improved her technique. She calculated her recommended weekly point total as follows:

She added these points:

| | |
|---|---|
| Good running form | 10 points |
| Ideal body weight | 10 points |

Points to add in Box A:  **20 points**

Then she subtracted these points:

| | |
|---|---|
| Current knee problems | 20 points |
| Knee pain after exercise | 20 points |

Points to subtract in Box B:  **40 points**

Her formula looks like this: **100 + 20 = 120 – 40 = 80 points.**

Now Julie does more of her running in the pool and less on the roads. She still competes **occasionally**, but not every weekend, as was her previous pattern. During weeks that she doesn't race, she runs more often, but even when she has a race, she stays under 80 points as in the program that follows:

| Monday | Run 7 miles on grass | 50 minutes | 10 points |
| | Stretch | 15 minutes | 0 points |
| Tuesday | Hike, some hills | 2 hours | 12 points |
| | Stretch | 30 minutes | 0 points |
| | Pool workout | 1 hour | 0 points |
| Wednesday | Run sprints on track | 1 hour | 12 points |
| | Pool workout | 1 hour | 0 points |
| Thursday | Run 6 miles on dirt | 42 minutes | 8 points |
| Friday | Pool workout | 90 minutes | 0 points |
| | Weight training—upper body | 30 minutes | 0 points |
| | Therapy exercises for knees | 15 minutes | 0 points |
| Saturday | Warm-up jog | 10 minutes | 3 points |
| | Stretch | 15 minutes | 0 points |
| | Road race 10K | 40 minutes | 10 points |
| Sunday | **Rest Day** | | |
| | Yoga: lying/sitting poses: | 1 hour | 3 points |
| | **Total Points:** | | <u>61</u> |

## Beach Volleyball sample

John played beach volleyball, all day, every Saturday and Sunday. He practiced his game at least once a week, rode his mountain bike, and golfed on the other days. At thirty-one, he'd had a knee arthroscopy (minor surgery) to trim out a small tear in his meniscus. At forty-two, the same knee began to bother him after workouts. He decided to be proactive and aggressively change his sports routine in an attempt to heal his knees. Here's his former weekly routine:

| | | | |
|---|---|---|---|
| Monday | Mountain bike | 90 minutes | **18 points** |
| | Stretch | 15 minutes | **0 points** |
| Tuesday | Volleyball practice games | 2 hours | **24 points** |
| | Stretch | 15 minutes | **0 points** |
| Wednesday | Golf—walking | 4 hours | **24 points** |
| Thursday | Volleyball practice games | 2 hours | **24 points** |
| Friday | Bike on bike path | 1 hour | **6 points** |
| Saturday | Stretch | 15 minutes | **0 points** |
| | Beach volleyball games | 3 hours | **36 points** |
| Sunday | Stretch | 15 minutes | **0 points** |
| | Beach volleyball games | 3 hours | **36 points** |
| | | **Total Points:** | <u>**168**</u> |

John calculated his weekly critical threshold like this:

He added these points:

| | | |
|---|---|---|
| | Good form during exercise | 10 points |
| | Ideal body weight | <u>10 points</u> |
| **Points to add in Box A:** | | **20 points** |

Points to subtract:

| | | |
|---|---|---|
| | Current knee problem | 20 points |
| | Knee pain after exercise | 20 points |
| | Previous knee surgery | <u>30 points</u> |
| **Points to subtract in Box B:** | | **70 points** |

John's formula is: **100 points +20 = 120 – 70 = 50 points**

John got serious about changing the impact he places on his knees. He cut back on the number of jumps he makes in the sand, he replaced his mountain bike with a road bike, and he rides in his golf cart instead of walking the course. He also substituted deep-water interval training (see page 162) for several hours of volleyball. He still enjoys his weekends at the beach, but he watches from his beach chair more often. This is his new program:

| Monday | **Rest Day** | | |
|---|---|---|---|
| | Stretch | 15 minutes | 0 points |
| | Therapy exercises for knees | 30 minutes | 0 points |
| Tuesday | Volleyball practice games | 1 hour | 12 points |
| | Pool workout | 1 hour | 0 points |
| | Stretch | 30 minutes | 0 point |
| Wednesday | Golf—riding in cart | 4 hours | 0 points |
| Thursday | Bike on bike path, some hills | 90 minutes | 9 points |
| | Stretch | 30 minutes | 0 point |
| Friday | Pool workout | 90 minutes | 0 points |
| | Therapy exercises for knees | 30 minutes | 0 points |
| Saturday | Beach volleyball games | 1 hour | 12 points |
| Sunday | Beach volleyball games | 1 hour | 12 points |
| | | **Total Points:** | <u>45</u> |

## EARLY WARNING SIGNS—INJURIES IN-THE-MAKING

If your knee complaint has been coming on for a long time, you may have developed a high tolerance for pain. You've learned to "live with it" and don't realize that you've begun to limp, not until a friend or a relative tells you. A limp is an early warning sign that something more serious is taking place in your knee. Other signs are swelling, stiffness, and decreased range of motion.

Harder to identify are warning signs that come from parts of your body other than your knee. Your natural tendency might be to have those painful areas—your hip or ankle or back—examined before considering another possibility: that your pain is the result of an altered gait caused by your sore knee.

---

**QUICKLY HEED EARLY WARNING SIGNS**

The majority of patients I see for osteoarthritis have damaged their knees in the past. I warn these patients who have had previous knee traumas or surgeries to be ultra conscientious in their choice of nurturing activities and heed early warning signs immediately. If you're medicating yourself to exercise, this may be an early warning sign.     —ROBERT KLAPPER, M.D.

---

Whatever your sport, there is a position, posture, stance, or alignment that helps the body perform smoothly and with the least effort. When you use correct biomechanics (good form), your movements are efficient and cause minimal jarring, tearing, or strain. Conversely, bad form— lack of correct biomechanics—can lead to increased strain and even to injury.

Runners, for instance, can create knee injuries with faulty biomechanics. Ask a fellow runner or a running coach to watch your form. Your knees should glide straight forward in front of you. Your feet should point straight forward and remain in line with your knees and hips at all times, never angling out to the side. Good arm action helps guide your leg action: swing your hands and elbows straight forward and backward to help force your knees and feet into better alignment. If your heels swing out to the sides, placing inward rotational torque on your knees, you have an injury in the making at every step. Stop now. Find a good coach to help you correct your form or switch to walking or one of the nurturing activities.

Whenever you exercise, aim at good form and ease of movement. Use pain and discomfort as your guide to know when you're moving incorrectly. By improving your form, you can often eliminate pain and be able to continue exercising.

## REST DAYS

If you are serious about fitness and your sports, you hate to be told you'll have to stop. But perhaps you are finally admitting that your knee isn't getting better, that it needs some rest.

Rest replenishes energy stores and rebuilds tissues damaged by continuous training. Rest is an integral part of every well-planned fitness program, for the body adapts to work stimulus **only if a rest period follows.** Knowing this, you must exert the same discipline in scheduling rest days as you do in planning workouts. Schedule one day of rest each week. On that day you can stretch if you find you must do **something** to alleviate nervous "twitchies" in muscles that are craving exercise. Generally, the older you are, the more recovery you need. If needed, schedule more than one day of rest a week.

## MANAGING INJURY AND RECOVERY

Stick with nurturing exercises until you are pain-free for more than a week before attempting your abusive sport again. If you feel pain when you return to your high-point activity, immediately return to the comfort of nurturing exercise. Use low-point activities to maintain your fitness while your injury heals. This time, wait until your knee is pain-free for at least two weeks before trying anything but nurturing exercises and the land therapy exercises in Chapter 11.

Don't be quick to take aspirin, Tylenol, Advil, Aleve, or any other painkillers. **Pain is your most important indicator of damage and can be a valuable guide for planning the recovery process.** Don't just make the pain go away: discover the reason for your pain and make **it** go away.

> **GOOD PAIN VS. BAD PAIN**
>
> Learn to differentiate between the good pain of training—muscles "burning" as they are stimulated to become stronger—and the bad pain of tendon injury or joint damage. You can often push through burning muscles, but you want to stop immediately upon feeling joint pain. Tendon pain is more complex: on days when sore tendons warm up and feel better with each passing minute, continue your workout; on days when tendons develop stabbing pains upon each step or muscle contraction, you must stop right away and ice the area.

## ANATOMICAL PREDISPOSITION TO KNEE INJURY

If you were blind, you wouldn't think of flying a plane. If you couldn't sink a foul shot, you'd be foolish to dream of playing professional basketball. And if your knee anatomy predisposes you to injury, it would likewise be foolish to take part in abusive activities. Let's say you've recently learned that you have the genetic abnormality called a discoid meniscus (see page 43). This meniscus is predisposed to meniscal tears, so you would want to avoid the twisting and pivoting of racquetball, football, basketball, and volleyball. You would also want to protect your knees from the high impact of running, aerobic classes, or stair climbing. Perhaps you've been teased all your life about being knock-kneed. You probably have patellar tracking difficulties, which means you're at risk for injuries to the meniscus or the kneecap. Avoid bouncing, jumping, and other high-impact activities.

If your knees bend more than average, they are said to hyperflex; if they straighten past the normal straight-leg position, they are said to hyperextend. These "hyper" knees are surrounded by lax (loose) ligaments that can be both a blessing and a curse. To visualize the "blessing," think of the willow tree that bends in a storm instead of a rigid oak that breaks. Ligament laxity in knees can help you survive traumatic incidents that would tear tighter knee structures. On the other hand, flexible knee joints can be a "curse" when they allow you to assume unusual positions (such as the cross-legged lotus pose in yoga) that can tear the meniscus or injure the kneecap.

If your kneecap doesn't track the way it should—straight down the center of the groove in your femur—you are anatomically predisposed to chondromalacia (see page 50). To prevent further damage to the cartilage on the back of your kneecap, eliminate abusive activities and strengthen the VMO (see page 50) to restore its ability to hold the kneecap in place.

Three factors determine your knee's stability:

1.  the laxity or tightness of the surrounding ligaments
2.  the bony anatomy where the tibia and femur meet
3.  the muscle tone of the surrounding muscles

**Although you can't do anything to change the ligaments or the bony anatomy, you *can* affect the muscles.** Powerful quadriceps, hamstrings, and calf muscles can function like shock absorbers in your car: they can absorb the jolts and bounces before such impact is transmitted to your knee joint. Stronger muscles mean safer knees, even if your knee anatomy is less than perfect.

## SELF TREATMENTS

A sudden injury that has just occurred, whether major or minor, is called an acute injury. Examples of acute injuries to the knee range from tendinitis during a long run to a torn ligament from a skiing fall to a ruptured patellar tendon when spiking a volleyball. You know immediately when such injuries occur because pain, swelling, and dysfunction accompany them. Bleeding takes place in the surrounding tissues, which causes sensitivity and pain in the nearby nerve endings. If the bleeding is major, a bruise will be created; when there's less bleeding in minor injuries, you may not see a bruise, but there will be some degree of bleeding, swelling, and pain. Minor acute injuries can seem an inconsequential part of post work-out soreness, but if left untreated, they can become chronic. You are said to have a chronic injury if the injury persists long after the standard six weeks required for tissue healing.

Learning to acknowledge the smallest injury to your knee and treating it immediately can stop more severe damage. Follow these steps when you feel an acute injury.

**REST:** Immediately stop doing the activity that caused the inflammation and let your knee rest until the pain has significantly diminished. Return to activity with **nurturing exercises only** until your knee has been pain-free at least a week.

**ICE:** Surround your knee with ice to prevent or diminish the expansion of the capillaries that leads to swelling. Apply ice for ten to twenty minutes, four to five times a day during the first forty-eight hours, then twice a day until the injury is resolved. If you don't have an ice pack, frozen peas mold nicely around knees. (See below and page 129 for more details on applying ice.)

### ICE MASSAGE

The knee joint is close to the surface, not buried beneath layers of muscles, so the therapeutic qualities of ice work quickly and well, especially with ice massage. Fill a paper cup with water and put it in the freezer. Once frozen, peel down the paper until about an inch of ice is exposed. What's left of the cup becomes a "handle" for this ice massage device. Begin making circular or back-and-forth motions with the ice cup on the sore areas of your knee. When your skin turns pink and feels numb, wrap your knee in a dry towel and enjoy the "thawing" sensation.

ELEVATION: Keep your knee raised to hold swelling to a minimum. Other self-help treatments for knee injuries appear in Chapter 7, pages 127 to 138.

## LIFELONG MANAGEMENT OF KNEE CONDITIONS

Maintaining an active lifestyle means **managing** your knee condition wisely and diligently. It means choosing nurturing exercises more often than you choose abusive exercises. With attention to the daily, weekly, and monthly condition of your knees, you **can** manage their care. You **can** prevent deterioration or injury. And you can take great joy from the days when your knees don't hurt. Those can be the days when you occasionally participate in your beloved sports and activities. Appreciate each hour your knees give you such pleasure, then reward them with a daily routine of nurturing exercise.

# 5 REACHING A DIAGNOSIS: DOING *YOUR* PART

Today you live in an information age when you can discover, with the click of a mouse, the latest developments in the diagnosis and treatment of medical conditions. This means you no longer need to rely solely on your doctors for medical knowledge. And by reading this book, you're now one of the many who is making an effort to understand your own knee problems.

---

**KNEE HELP ON THE WEB**
Keep up with the latest research on new knee treatments and check regularly the latest information we make available on our Web site, www.kneehelp.com. There you'll find photos of the latest pool and land exercises as well as case studies of former patients who have successfully healed their knees.

---

## A WRITTEN PHYSICAL HISTORY

A good way to continue delving for information is to prepare a physical history. Use the form that follows to trigger your thinking. Go over each item carefully, and as you do, you'll probably surprise yourself by remembering events from years ago. You may also think of details not included on the form. Write them down. Begin to keep track day by day of your pain: what part of your knee hurts and how often, what time of day your knee seems to hurt most, and what kinds of things you do that aggravate and relieve the pain.

People often say, "All I did was bend to pick a flower. How could I have hurt myself so badly?" The answer is that if you think back six or eight weeks, you'll probably remember changing your exercise routine or helping someone move heavy boxes. You probably tore ninety-five percent of a muscle, tendon, ligament, or meniscus at that time but had no symptoms. Then, two months later, a minor twisting movement caused the other five percent of the structure to tear. With such lag time between the inciting event and knee pain, your job becomes that of a dectective. Dig back into the past. It's easy to forget a blow to your knee from a frisky dog, a trip off a curb, or a stumble up some stairs if no pain resulted. Yet most of the injury could have been caused at that earlier time.

Don't overlook a remembered pain that was once acute but then vanished and never returned. To understand how this could have happened, consider an analogy: A woman starts a new gardening activity that strenuously uses her hands and develops a blister on her palm that causes acute pain. She gives the blister a few days to heal, then continues gardening off and on over the next months. The blister eventually turns into a callus, the pain completely deadened. Your earlier pain could have disappeared in that same way. Remembering such a previous flare-up of knee pain can greatly help in diagnosing your condition.

## PHYSICAL HISTORY

What is your knee problem?

    Pain ____

    Limping, but no pain ____

    Giving way ____

    Locking ____

    Unstable ____

    Faulty gait or walking pattern ____

    Limited movement ____

        Doesn't bend all the way ____

        Doesn't straighten all the way ____

    Baker cyst ____

    Tendon(s) ____

    Ligament(s) ____

    Meniscus(i) ____

What is the location of your pain: (Circle all that apply.)

| | L = Left | R = right | B = Both |
|---|---|---|---|
| Front of knee | L | R | B |
| Back of knee | L | R | B |
| Inner side of knee | L | R | B |
| Outer side of knee | L | R | B |
| Below knee cap | L | R | B |
| Above knee cap | L | R | B |
| Shin | L | R | B |
| Calf | L | R | B |
| Foot | L | R | B |

When did the pain start?

    After trauma ____

    After a heavy workout ____

    After a fall ____

    Gradual onset with no specific beginning date ____

    Other, explain

_____

_____

Have you had a problem with your knees in the past?

    As a child ____

    As a teenager ____

    Previous trauma ____  Explain _____

    Previous surgery ____  Explain _____

    New problem ____

    Other, explain _____

    _____

Is your knee problem associated with work or exercises you're doing?

_____

_____

Have you begun any new sports or activities?

    Aerobics ____

    Basketball ____

    Kickboxing ____

    Martial arts ____

    Racquetball ____

    Running ____

    Skiing ____

    Soccer ____

    Stair climbing ____

    Volleyball ____

    Other(s) _____

Do you have any new sports injuries? Please describe:

_____

Do you have any old sports injuries? Please describe:

_____

What relieves the pain? _____

_____

What makes the pain worse? _____
_____

What medications are you currently taking? (Please include aspirin,
over-the-counter medications, herbs, homeopathics, birth control pills,
hormones, vitamins, food supplements, etc.)
_____

Have you taken any new medications in the last year?
_____

Have you had prior treatment, tests, or diagnoses on your knee(s)?
    In the past year ____
    Many years ago ____
    Please be specific _____
_____

What have you done for the pain?
    Nothing yet ____
    Visiting doctor ____
    Taken prescription anti-inflammatories ____
    Taken anti-inflammatories (aspirin, Motrin, Advil) ____
    Changed fitness routine ____
    Stopped exercising ____
    Wearing a knee brace or wrap (now or in the past) ____
    Using a cane ____
    Using a walker ____
    Using a wheelchair ____

Have you had injections into your knee joint? If so, how many and when?
    Cortisone _____
    Synvisk _____

Do you have a family history of knee problems? ____ Yes ____ No

Has your environment changed in the past year?
    Started working ＿＿
    Stopped working ＿＿
    Changed jobs ＿＿
    Moved to a new home ＿＿
    House has more stairs ＿＿
    Office has more stairs ＿＿

Have you moved to a new climate?
    Moved from humid climate to dry ＿＿
    Moved from dry climate to humid ＿＿

Have you begun wearing new shoes or orthotics? Explain:

_____

_____

Are you exercising on a different type of terrain (grass, dirt, asphalt)?

_____

_____

Have you had recent surgery or pain involving other parts of your body?

_____

_____

How is the rest of your health? _____

_____

Have you had recent weight changes?
    Loss of ＿＿ pounds in the past ＿＿ months
    Gain of ＿＿ pounds in the past ＿＿ months
    No change in weight ＿＿

Has anything changed in your driving habits?
    New car ＿＿
    Longer commute ＿＿
    Shorter commute ＿＿

Have you had a recent increase in travel?

    Increased air travel ___

    Increased car travel ___

    Increased train travel ___

Have you changed your diet? If so, how _____

_____

Are you having trouble with your activities of daily living?

    Walking ___

    Going up and down stairs ___

    Getting in and out of the car ___

    Getting up and down from a sofa or chair ___

    Other, list _____

## The Home Self-Examination

Once you've completed your written history, stand facing a full-length mirror for a self-examination. Wear a bathing suit or shorts so you can see the full length of both legs. Breathe comfortably and relax until you feel you are standing as you normally would.

NOTICE THE ALIGNMENT OF YOUR LEGS. Are they straight up and down? Are you bowlegged—meaning your knees are bowed out while your ankles are close together? Are you knock-kneed, meaning that your knees are close together but your ankles are far apart? People who are bowlegged tend to develop osteoarthritis in the medial (inner) compartment of the knee, because their stance doesn't distribute the body's weight evenly across both the medial and lateral compartments but overloads just the medial portion. People who are knock-kneed overload the lateral (outer) part of the knee, are more likely to tear the lateral meniscus, and often have the patella tracking problems discussed on page 50.

CHECK THE ORIENTATION OF YOUR FEET. Do your feet roll inward? If one or both feet drop inward toward the floor, they are said to pronate, which makes you more knock-kneed. Do your feet roll outward? If so, they are said to supinate or drop outward, which makes you more bow-legged. Excessive pronation or supination can lead to foot problems which, in turn, can cause ankle and knee problems as the faulty mechanical forces are transmitted upward. Faulty orientation of your feet may be the cause of your knee cap pain, joint pain, tendinitis, or other knee complaints.

---

**ORTHOTICS**

Podiatrists will often suggest putting orthotic inserts into your shoes to help correct the alignment of your foot. These orthotics sometimes allow you to load your weight more evenly on both compartments of your knee joint, and for people with patello-femoral pain, they can be a good first step toward resolving the pain. In my opinion, however, orthotics are overutilized— they're suggested to many more people than actually need them.　　　　　　　　　　　　　—DR. ROBERT KLAPPER

---

ARE YOU STANDING STRAIGHT OR ARE YOU LEANING? Do you have most of your weight on one leg? If you've previously had knee trauma or surgery, you may have unconsciously adjusted your normal stance to take your weight off a sore knee. Such an adjustment may have taken place in your walking pattern as well. Write this down to tell your doctor and ask him or her to check your gait.

---

**LEG-LENGTH DISCREPANCY**

Be skeptical when someone says, "All of your problems come from your leg length." Everyone has a slight difference in the size of their hands, their feet, and the length of their legs. If you have less than a ¼-inch difference in leg lengths, your body has probably already adjusted. If you put a lift in your shoe, you may be robbing Peter to pay Paul, because you could be creating a lower back problem.

---

ARE YOUR KNEES SWOLLEN? Patients often point to one spot and say, "It's only swollen right here." But your knee has a bony patella in front, so when the joint fills with fluid it doesn't fill symmetrically like a beach ball. Your entire knee may be swollen, but your kneecap is preventing swelling in the anterior, or front, of the knee.

When does your knee swell: After exercise? After you've been on your feet a while? When you wake up? At the end of the day? If your knee swells when you've been vertical a while, but when you rest and elevate your leg the swelling dissipates, that tells you the vascular pathways that return blood from your leg to your heart are working but that they are overloaded. If the swelling doesn't come down overnight when you're lying down, that points to a more acute injury. Perhaps you broke a blood vessel in one of the ligaments inside the knee joint. Or maybe there's an infection in your knee that's causing the swelling. Writing down when your knee swells and how long it stays swollen can provide you and your doctor with valuable information.

TURN SIDEWAYS TO SEE IF YOU CAN BEND AND STRAIGHTEN YOUR KNEES COMPLETELY. Lift one heel toward your buttocks and make a mental note of its height. Bend the other knee and see if that heel rises to the same height as the other foot. Next, see if both knees straighten to the same position. Does one knee stop moving before it is fully straight? If one knee doesn't bend as far as the other, or if one can't fully straighten, make note of this in your physical history under "limited movement." Do your knees hyperextend? That is, do they move beyond a straight line into a backward curve? People with loose ligaments around their knees can straighten them past the normal position. There's nothing wrong with having knees that hyperextend, as long as both knees are the same. If one knee hyperextends and the other doesn't, point that out to your doctor for further investigation.

FEEL THE BACK OF YOUR KNEES. About fifteen percent of the human population have a Baker cyst behind the knee (see page 55). If you've had a Baker cyst all your life, check to see if it's become more pronounced than usual. Increased fluid going into your Baker cyst may indicate other problems in the knee.

FEEL THE SIDES OF YOUR KNEES. If you feel a bulge on either side of your knee, you may have a meniscal cyst (see page 54), which means there's a tear in the meniscus on that side of your knee.

GET DRESSED AND GO UP AND DOWN SOME NEARBY STAIRS. Are you able to reciprocate the stairs; that is, are you able to put your right foot on one step, your left foot on the next step, and continue in that manner? Or are you putting your right foot on a step, then putting your left foot on the same step in order to advance? A fit knee is able to reciprocate going both upstairs and downstairs. Losing the ability to reciprocate stairs is one of the first changes in your gait you'll notice if your knee is unfit. If you cannot perform this activity of daily living, tell your doctor during the exam.

INSPECT THE WAY YOUR SHOES ARE WEARING. Your shoes are like the tires on your car; they can tell you if your alignment is off. So notice if there's a difference between one shoe and the other. Go to your closet and compare the soles of several  pairs of new and old shoes. Notice if you're wearing through your newer shoes faster and in a pattern different from your usual wear pattern. This subtle difference could be an early indicator of arthritic changes in your knee.

## SEEKING HELP FROM A DOCTOR

Now that you've completed the written history and the self-exam, and taken time to consider your answers, you are prepared to help your doctor diagnose and treat your unfit knee—that is, if you've decided to consult a doctor. Your reason for doing so may be as hard to describe as your "sixth sense." Or your reasons may depend entirely on the strength and duration of your pain, the restriction of your daily activities because of the soreness of your knee joint, or the alteration of your gait—at some point along the continuum of knee symptoms, you'll decide to seek relief by combining your knowledge with a doctor's.

What kind of doctor you see may be determined by what kind of health insurance you carry. You may be required to see a general practitioner before you can visit a specialist such as an orthopedist, a primary care doctor for the musculoskeletal system who offers a range of surgical procedures and nonsurgical therapies to treat your knee. If your insurance allows you to choose any doctor directly, keep this in mind: The kind of doctor you visit is the kind of medicine you'll get. In other words, if you go to a surgeon, he or she may be biased toward surgery and drugs. If you visit a physiatrist, a medical doctor who specializes in rehabilitation, you'll be guided toward medical techniques such as anti-inflammatories, injections, and rehabilitative exercise. If you choose a rheumatologist, you'll find medical but not surgical treatments for arthritis and connective tissue diseases, such as osteoarthritis, rheumatoid arthritis, lupus, and gout. A trip to the chiropractor brings nonsurgical, nondrug treatments such as manipulations, exercise, ultrasound, and electrotherapy treatments. Physical therapists offer joint and soft-tissue mobilization (passive movement), ice/heat, electrotherapy treatments and therapeutic exercise on land and in a pool. In some states you're allowed direct access to physical therapists, meaning you can go directly to the therapist for treatment. Other states require that you obtain a prescription for physical therapy from an M.D. If your tendency is to stay away from Western medicine, consider the alternative medicine treatments such as acupuncture, herbs, homeopathies, and others, discussed in Chapter 7.

---

### THE BEST INFORMATION

It's always appropriate to get a second opinion about your condition. Each health-care provider has a bias toward certain procedures, and you'll want to hear several points of view in order to make the best possible choice for the care of your knee.

---

Do your research to find the best knee doctor in your area. Use the Internet, talk to friends and relatives who speak highly of their doctors, and use books such as *Top Doctors*, which lists the doctors other doctors go to when they need health care. Once you've found your top choice, be prepared to wait. The best doctors are usually worth waiting for.

Schedule an appointment and take along your written physical history for discussion during your initial office visit. I've summarized the possible implications of your history in the pages that follow.

**FORM POSITIVE RELATIONSHIPS WITH YOUR DOCTOR'S STAFF**

- Treat the staff with the same respect you show the doctor. They, too, are health-care professionals, from the person who schedules your appointments to the X ray technician to the person calling your insurance company for authorization. Learn their names. Be gracious. You'll have a more satisfying, overall experience.
- Understand how busy most doctors' offices are and be as concise as possible when making your first call for an appointment. Save your symptoms and the details about your knee for the doctor.
- If you're in pain and you're having trouble getting an appointment right away, ask to speak to the office manager. Pain is graded on a scale of 1 to 10. If your pain level is 8 or above, tell the office manager that, and he or she will probably squeeze you in the same week. Ask what you can do to help yourself until your appointment. Never exaggerate your pain or the urgency of your case, because once you're examined, if your condition or pain level didn't require a rush, you will not have endeared yourself to the staff.

## Symptoms

How long have you had knee problems? Weeks? Months? Did the problem start suddenly or come on gradually? Is the pain associated with an acute event, an accident or an injury, or has it been a slowly progressive problem? The location of the pain and the length of time it has existed will help in making a correct diagnosis.

> **EMERGENCIES**
>
> If something severe has just happened to your knee, the criteria below will help you determine if your condition is an emergency:
> - Your knee is locked.
> - Your knee is swollen and hot—you suspect it could be infected.
> - You've broken a bone.
> - Your knee is dislocated.
>
> These are all clear-cut orthopedic emergencies. Tell the office manager that your case is an emergency.

## Exacerbating Factors

When you've been sitting in your car, on an airplane, or in a chair at the movies or in a restaurant, do you feel a sharp pain behind the patella when you stand and take your first steps? This is called starting pain and is considered pathognomonic to patellofemoral problems. Pathognomonic symptoms are the equivalent of a bull's-eye, the real signal that indeed you have a problem in your patellofemoral joint and not elsewhere.

Picture an auto mechanic in a small-town gas station. As you drive your car in, it's making a noise, and from across the garage the mechanic says, "It's your intake manifold, and spark plug number four needs to be changed." He hears in the way the car is idling what's wrong. The sound is pathognomonic to him. That's what starting pain is to patellofemoral problems.

Does your knee hurt when you go up and down stairs? That, too, is an indicator of patellofemoral problems. Although more people say their knees hurt going downstairs than upstairs, you can experience knee pain moving in either direction.

Does your favorite workout or sport make your knee sore? Does the pain go away when you cut back on your recreational activities?

Do you have knee pain after walking a certain length of time? When you sit down does the pain go away?

Answers to these questions will tell whether this is a circulatory or neurological problem. If your knee pain worsens as you walk but goes away completely when you sit down, that can indicate a circulatory problem. If, however, the pain in your knee gets worse as you walk, but it does not go away when you sit to rest, that may indicate a neurological condition such as a herniated disk or a pinched nerve.

When you have pain in and around your knee, its source is usually the knee; however, make sure your doctor does a thorough exam to determine that your knee pain is coming from your knee and not your hip or lower back.

## Medications

Discuss with your doctor the medications and supplements you are currently taking: prescription drugs, aspirin and other over-the-counter pain relievers, hormone replacement, wellness supplements, amino acids, calcium, herbs, homeopathics, vitamin C, multivitamins, and birth control pills. Are you having side effects? Do you know which medicine or supplement is causing which effect?

Some people feel better taking over-the-counter anti-inflammatories such as Advil, Tylenol, and aspirin, while others feel better taking the new oral prescription medications called Cox II Inhibitors (Vioxx, Celebrex, and Bextra). What both categories of drugs share is that they have significant side effects, and you should be careful using any of them. The new drugs have brought with them cardiac symptoms we never saw before, so I believe that their side effects are worse.

**REFRAIN FROM INJECTIONS**

- Anytime a needle is placed into your knee joint, you run the risk of infection or of synovitis, which is an inflammation of the joint's lining.
- Drug companies are touting the benefits of new medicines to be injected into the knee that can help grow cartilage. They don't really grow cartilage and the risks involved aren't yet known.
- Avoid cortisone injections, because cortisone is very disruptive to the articular cartilage. Although it's a short-term solution to take away inflammation, the medication lingers in the joint, corroding your crucial cartilage.

## Prior Treatment

Have you seen another doctor or therapist previously for this knee condition? If so, have you followed his or her suggestions? Have you had previous therapy, tests, or diagnoses? Have you had previous knee surgery or fractures? Did you have knee problems in childhood?

If you had surgery in childhood and an infection developed in any of the bones near your knee, that would be important to know, even if the infection was treated successfully. That infection may have destroyed some of the bone or the growth plate at the end of the bone, destruction that can lead to problems later on. If you have a poor recollection of your childhood, talk to your parents, siblings, or other relatives. If any of them have memories of your having had surgery or wearing a brace as a child, you owe it to yourself to get an X ray. Then you will know the status of your knee.

In the more recent past, you may have seen various doctors or therapists for your ongoing knee problem. One doctor's solution to a problem in the past may now be the cause of your current knee problem. If you can assemble all the previous information you have gathered about your knee to give to your current doctor, you and the doctor won't have to start the learning process all over again. Do your best to understand the conclusions other doctors have reached in order to summarize them during your conversation with your new doctor.

---

**ATTENTION HMO USERS**

If your knee hurts and you've waited over a month for it to get better but it hasn't, you absolutely need an X ray. What you're feeling might be a symptom of something bigger. You want to rule out a fracture, a dislocation, or a tumor. It's not a waste of time or money; it is necessary for a thorough exam. But if you're my patient and you twisted your leg, heard a pop, and your knee is swollen, I'll often skip most of the manual tests of the initial exam, because they would inflict too much pain. You've probably torn your ACL, but I won't know for sure until I see the MRI. So we skip the X ray and get an MRI. Why go through pain to find out what the MRI will tell? Don't let an HMO short change you and cause you pain.                    —ROBERT KLAPPER, M.D.

---

## Functional Assessment

How well you function in everyday life is considered your functional capacity. Are you currently performing your activities of daily living despite the problems you're having with your knee? Can you walk up and downstairs? Can you get in and out of a car? Can you do the duties required of you in your work or home responsibilities? Do you need a knee brace, a wrap, or a cane to move smoothly throughout the day?

How well do you walk? Do you limp or shorten your steps? If you're limping it's because of knee pain or weakness of the quadriceps and hamstring muscles.

---

**OBSERVATIONS OF DAILY KNEE LIFE**

I watch my patients move around the office so I can have a glimpse of what their daily knee life is like. I watch how quickly or slowly they move and how they get up from the chair. Do they grimace in pain as they stand up? I watch these things not because patients might be hiding something from me, but because I can sometimes see more in their movements than they can see themselves. They've made lifestyle changes, adaptations of movement that they can no longer notice.

---

## The Doctor's Physical Exam

When a patient comes into my office complaining of knee pain, the first thing I do is examine the other knee. If both knees hurt, I start my exam with the most normal knee. This is a time for me to go slowly so I can discover what's normal for this patient's knees. If the normal knee is loose, I won't think there's ligament damage if the sore knee is equally loose. If one knee hyperextends, I won't consider it a problem when I examine the painful knee. Only when one side is different from the other have I found something to look into.

I perform a series of tests that give me an indication of what could be happening in the knee. Are the ligaments and menisci intact? Is the patellofemoral joint the culprit? Are the tendons injured? The sounds and sensations related to this knee offer me information to interpret in the context of thousands of other knee exams I've already performed.

**THE KNEE EXAM SHOULDN'T BE PAINFUL**

Your doctor should perform each test on your knee very gently. That way, if he stimulates the problem area, you'll feel only the slightest twinge of pain. If you're apprehensive about any part of the exam, tell your doctor—your uneasiness may help locate the trouble spot. After the exam, you shouldn't be in pain.

Listed below are the items I check in sequence on each knee patient.

**LOOK AND FEEL FOR SWELLING.** In a thin or average-size person, knee anatomy is fairly easy to see and feel. In patients who are obese, it's more difficult. I put my hand over each knee to feel for heat or swelling. If I find swelling, this is the most nonspecific piece of information I collect— it simply tells me something is wrong with the joint and that the lining is inflamed. As I perform the rest of the exam, I'll try to determine whether the knee is inflamed because of a mechanical problem, a recent injury, an infection, or a chronic condition such as gout or rheumatoid arthritis. If the cause of swelling is due to trauma, we'll begin treatments such as those outlined in Chapter 7. If it seems as though something more systemic is occurring in the body, I'll aspirate the knee. That is, I'll withdraw fluid from the knee joint to send to the lab. If crystals are found, that implies gout. If a culture of the joint fluid grows bacteria, that means infection. If I suspect rheumatoid arthritis, I'll order a blood test.

**ASSESS OVERALL ALIGNMENT.** I look at the overall alignment of both legs. I want to see if the patient is at risk for developing certain problems because of poor alignment of the knees or, conversely, if he or she may have developed bad alignment because an old hip or ankle injury has taken its toll on the knees. If I see that the patient is bowlegged, my first concern will be that she may have worn out the medial meniscus and is now developing osteoarthritis in the medial compartment of the knee. If I find she's knock-kneed, there are three concerns: that she may have worn out the lateral meniscus and is getting OA in the lateral compartment, that she has a patella tracking problem, or that she's at risk for having her kneecap dislocate. If the knees are well-aligned, that's great news, because alignment is the knee's main Rock of Gibraltar.

MEASURE RANGE OF MOTION OF THE KNEES AND HIPS. I ask the patient to bend and straighten both knees and hips so I can check his or her range of motion. Can the knee fully bend and straighten? Is the knee so inflamed or full of fluid that it can't bend? Is there a torn ligament or a loose piece of meniscus blocking the joint from reaching full extension? Do bone spurs or other deformities of osteoarthritis inside the joint keep it from smoothly bending and straightening? Do the hips move freely through their normal full range of motion, or does a limitation in that joint affect the way the knees move?

FEEL PATELLAR TRACKING DURING FLEXION AND EXTENSION. I place my hand on the patient's knee as I bend and straighten it to feel how the knee cap tracks. Is the knee cap the source of the knee pain? Do I feel crepitus; that is, does the knee grind or creak as I move it? The amount of crepitus in a joint is usually an indicator of how much damage has occurred to the cartilage. Orthopedists grade arthritic changes in joints on a standard scale from 0 to 4. If I feel movement that is smooth, like two ice cubes rubbing together, that is 0 crepitus (no arthritis). A mild amount of grinding is a grade 1, while a noisy knee that sounds like crunching a bag of potato chips is a 4.

CHECK STABILITY—SIDE TO SIDE. As I check the stability of the knee, both side-to-side and front-to-back, I'm trying to find out if the ligaments are intact. First I stabilize the thigh with one hand and hold the Achilles tendon with the other. I use my hands as a brace, then apply slight sideways pressure, attempting to open the knee outward. If it moves more than the normal amount, or if the patient feels tenderness while I do this, it probably indicates an injured medial collateral ligament (MCL). Next I apply gentle sideways pressure to try to bend the knee inward. If it moves beyond the norm or if it is tender, it can indicate an injured lateral collateral ligament (LCL).

CHECK STABILITY—FRONT TO BACK. To check the anterior cruciate ligament (ACL) and the posterior crucial ligament (PCL), I bend the patient's knee so the foot is flat on the table, then I pull gently on the lower leg as if opening a drawer. The lower leg will move dramatically forward in a knee with a torn ACL. For the PCL test, I move the lower leg backward as though closing a drawer. If torn, it will move much more than the movement possible in a fit knee.

PERFORM PALPATION OF JOINT LINE, WITH KNEE BENT TO 90 DEGREES. I will feel along the joint line of the knee. If the patient feels piercing pain as I palpate the medial side of the knee, that probably indicates damage to the medial meniscus. If there's sharp pain as I probe the lateral side of the joint line, there's probably damage to the lateral meniscus.

LOOK FOR MENISCUS PAIN DURING ROTATION. Sometimes patients don't feel meniscus tenderness when I feel along the joint line because the tear isn't in the anterior horn, the front of the knee. When I try to probe along the back of the knee, the muscles are thicker there and it's harder to detect meniscus pain. So if the meniscus is torn in the posterior horn, I will have to rotate the knee to find the pain of the injury. This has to be done very gently. I place one hand on the heel of the patient's foot and stabilize their thigh with my other hand. If the meniscus is torn in the back of the knee, the patient will grimace in pain as I twist. Sometimes I'll hear a pop as the meniscus flops in and out of position. The patient will feel both instability and pain during rotation.

### KNEE PAIN CAN COME FROM YOUR HIP

While it's extremely unusual for patients who have bad knees to be feeling pain in their hips, it often happens that patients with bad hips have knee pain. Here's my theory on why this happens: the big quadriceps muscles that run down the front of the thigh have four muscles in that group. The rectus femoris, one of the most powerful of the four muscles, has an anchoring site close to the front of the hip joint capsule. If there's heat or pain in the hip joint, it can radiate down the whole rectus femoris muscle (see illustration 5-1). This means that patients who have an inflamed hip joint capsule often feel deep pain down the fronts of their thighs and are misled into thinking they have a knee problem instead of a hip problem.

**5-1**
The head of the rectus femoris muscle near the hip can cause radiating pain down to the knee.

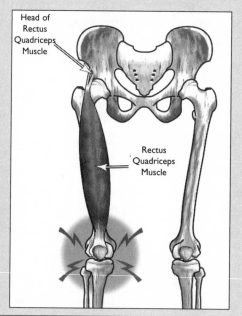

Head of
Rectus
Quadriceps
Muscle

Rectus
Quadriceps
Muscle

## Hips, Ankles, and Back

Besides checking a patient's knees, I also look at the hips, ankles, and back. Pain, swelling, and limited movement in those joints can create poor gait mechanics that can lead to knee problems. Knee pain can be due to a hip problem (see figure 5-1), due to a pinched nerve in the back, or bad walking patterns created from a sore ankle. While swelling isn't obvious around the hip or the back, it is clearly visible at the ankles. If the ankles are swollen, it could mean that a problem in the knee is disrupting the normal blood flow to and from the ankles, or there may be a systemic condition such as lupus, rheumatoid arthritis, or a heart problem.

## Neurological Exam

The human body has two kinds of nerves: sensory and motor. The sensory nerves transmit sensations from the body to the brain so you know what your body is feeling. The motor nerves transmit your intention to move from the brain to the muscles, causing movement. I test both sets of nerves. First, I test the foot's ability to register light touch and deep touch. A different set of nerve fibers registers light touch and deep touch, so I test both. I brush a piece of paper on the patient's foot to see if she feels it. If she doesn't, I could be picking up an early indication of diabetes. For deep touch, I apply pressure with my fingers on the top of the foot and ask the patient if she can feel it. Then I repeat the procedure on the bottom of the foot. I also check to see if the patient has sensation in the tips of her toes. After I've checked the sensory nerves, I test the motor nerves. I'll ask the patient to pull her foot upward and resist me as I try to push the foot down. Then I'll ask her to do the opposite movement, as though she were pushing down on a gas pedal. Again, I'll provide resistance and lift up against the force. If one leg is working well and the other isn't, we can probably assume nerve problems rather than muscle weakness.

## Pulses

There are two areas in the foot and ankle that represent the overall circulation to the big vessels of the lower extremities. We grade these pulses either Grade 0, Grade 1+, or Grade 2+. The dorsalis pedis pulse is on the top of the foot. The posterior tibial pulse is behind the inner ankle bone, called the medial malleolus. If your pulse is absent, you're probably not a candidate for surgery and you'll need to focus on rehabilitation through exercise. If you and your doctor feel you need surgery to correct your knee anatomy, a vascular surgeon could do noninvasive vascular studies to evaluate the integrity of the blood vessels. Without viable circulation, you would be at tremendous risk for surgery.

## Additional Tests

Should your doctor feel he needs more information to help diagnose your knee condition, he may order an MRI or a CT scan, which are discussed in the next chapter.

# 6 X RAYS, MRIs, AND CT SCANS

Objective tests are the universal language of medicine. I could be in China and unable to converse with another doctor, but as soon as we look at a set of X rays, we would both be able to see what was happening in a knee joint. Similarly, once you learn the basics of looking at your X ray, MRI, or CT scan, you will begin to understand knowledge that is shared universally. In this chapter, we hope to give you the means to explain your knee complaints more clearly to your doctor and better understand his or her diagnosis.

Figure 6-1A shows an X ray of a normal knee from the front while Figure 6-1B shows the same knee from the side. You'll return to these X rays several times as you read this chapter.

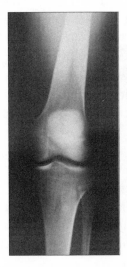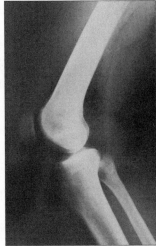

**6-1A**
The front view of a normal knee. Notice the smooth surfaces on both sides of the joint. The dark space between those two surfaces is cartilage.

**6-1B**
The side view of a normal knee. Notice the patella at the front of the joint. The femur is the thigh bone at the top; the tibia is the larger of the two bones in the lower leg; the fibula is the smaller.

In the classic teachings of medical school, there are subjective complaints of the patient, and objective findings such as this X ray. The subjective complaints are things you tell your doctor about where your knee hurts, how badly and frequently it hurts, and when the pain began. Although this information is crucial to helping your doctor reach a diagnosis, it isn't tangible—you can't see it or touch it. But an X ray is tangible, an objective finding you can actually see. So is an MRI and a CT Scan. All three tests offer different kinds of information.

A radiologist is a medical doctor who has been certified as a specialist in interpreting imaging studies such as X rays, MRIs and CT scans. Orthopedists and other physicians often consult with a radiologist for interpretation of the more complicated findings that appear on these imaging studies. It takes years of training and experience to be able to read an X ray, MRI, or CT Scan, so our goal certainly isn't to make you a radiologist, only to demystify a complicated area of medicine. This real knowledge can help you visualize your knee problem, understand your options for treatment, and assume responsibility for healing.

These days, state-of-the-art imaging centers use a digital PACS, which stands for Picture Archiving and Communications System. Think of how your home digital camera stores pictures on a disk, yet you can print them onto photo paper if you wish. The PACS works in the same way: digital information from a filmless radiology system is stored at a digital archive, yet can be printed onto plain film or burned onto a CD for your doctor. The PACS takes the images, then instead of spitting out an X ray or MRI sheet of film, transmits the data over an Ethernet cable to a work station in the imaging center for immediate viewing by the radiologist. Your study can be burned onto a CD disk and sent to your doctor for viewing on any desktop or laptop computer. The doctor slips the CD into his or her computer to see the images and follow along with the report. You'll no longer need to carry a packet of films that can so easily be lost or damaged. (PACS images can also be viewed on the Internet, just the way you access and view photo albums with family and friends.)

---

**NEW TECHNOLOGY: STUDIES ARE NEVER LOST**

Until recently, when you had your X rays taken, that original film was the only information that linked you to your exam. If it was lost or destroyed, it was as if that study was never done, because those films could not be brought back—your history was gone. Today, if you lose or break your CD, we can burn you a new one, because your information is not stored exclusively where your study was taken—it is also stored in backup locations (digital archives) around the country in case a fire or other catastrophe strikes an imaging center.

—RADIOLOGIST DOUGLAS H. BROWN, M.D.

---

**INTERCHANGEABLE INFORMATION WORLDWIDE**

PACS systems are available all over the world, but in far greater numbers in the United States and Western Europe. Most major American universities decided to switch to digital imagining in the late 1990s and are now operating on various PACS systems, all of which are compatible with each other. So if a patient brings a CD from New York, or even Pakistan, where she had an MRI three years ago and wants me to compare it with the new MRI she had today at our center, we can load images from the CD onto our computer and bring up the two imaging studies side by side for comparison. I can also download her old MRI into our system for storage and future access.         —RADIOLOGIST DOUGLAS H. BROWN, M.D.

Some doctors prefer studies on sheets of film for viewing on a light box as they discuss the results with their patients. Other doctors or hospitals haven't yet phased out their old film machines because of the time, effort, and major cost involved in switching to digital. So if your doctor orders an X ray or MRI for your knee, ask if he or she would like the information on a CD, plain film, or both.

Radiologists can manipulate digital images in several key ways to see more clearly into your knee as they look for the cause of your pain: they can enlarge the image, and they can alter the contrast and the brightness. The resolution on the PACS workstation is excellent, allowing radiologists to enlarge the image to double or triple its original size without losing clarity. Let's say we want to measure the thickness of a knee's cartilage. It will be easier to take that measurement on an enlarged image than on a smaller image. If your study was done on plain film, once that film is printed from an old-style X ray machine, that's all you've got to work with. Digitally acquired images, however, give the people reading those images much more power in manipulating them for accurate measurements and interpretations.

Another way to manipulate a PACS image is to change its window (contrast) and level (brightness), just as you would on a TV or on a computer monitor. When a doctor gets printed film, its window and level are designated by the machine or the technologist at that time. If the films are too light or too dark, there's nothing the doctor can do about it, and he consequently may not be able to see the damage in the knee. But if the films are done on PACS, the window and level can be altered on the work station to make the contrast sharper and the images darker or lighter, based on the preferences of the person reading the study. For example, when looking for a meniscal tear on an MRI study of the knee, the tear can be brought out more discreetly as a white line through a black meniscus.

Technological advances have been rapid in the field of imaging. Outside of the universities, however, most imaging centers are trying to catch up. Many hospitals have begun the move to digital, but it's often incomplete for technical and monetary reasons. They may have eighty percent of their systems switched to digital, but that leaves twenty percent using the old-style, film-only machines. In outpatient imaging away from universities or hospitals, there's an even greater lag in technological upgrades.

Your orthopedic surgeon will probably have his own X ray machine, but if an MRI or CT scan is required, you'll most likely be sent elsewhere for those images. Even if your doctor refers you to his favorite imaging center, call to make sure they have a PACS system with the ability to burn your study to a CD or print film according to your doctor's preference. If they don't, find a PACS nearby. If you live in a small town or rural area, it will be worth your travel time to the nearest university to obtain a modern study that lets you store your life-long health history in a form that is more secure and more adjustable for present and future interpretation. The most advanced technology offers you the best possibility of finding the cause of your pain, because once you have a PACS study on CD, you can go to another doctor or radiologist for a second opinion. The new doctor can manipulate images to his or her own preferences for careful inspection.

No matter where your studies are taken, it's important for you to look at your X rays and MRIs with your doctor, not to settle for the radiologist's report. This is the time for you to learn about your own knee.

**If you might be pregnant, you should avoid having an X ray, MRI, or CT Scan. Before you have any of these tests, you'll be asked a series of questions in advance that will ensure your safety.**

## X RAYS

X rays use electromagnetic radiation to penetrate solids and create gray-scale images. These images give doctors a look at parts of the body that have density, such as calcium. Bones have calcium, so we see them on X rays, which are an indispensable tool in the orthopedic examination of a patient, exposing a fracture, dislocation, tumor, or other pathologic changes.

Let's suppose you have a normal knee and a problematic knee. Look again at the X rays of the normal knee on page 115. You can see where the femur and tibia meet, but on the X ray they're not touching each other. The space between them isn't air, it's the cartilage at the end of your bones, but because cartilage doesn't have calcium, it doesn't show up on the X ray.

When you see that space on an X ray, you can conclude there's a healthy cartilage space between the femur and tibia. The joint is normal. Now when you look at a degenerating knee and see the femur getting closer to the tibia, that means a loss of joint space, a loss of the cartilage, which generally means degenerative arthritis. Notice in Figure 6-2A that the joint space has narrowed in the medial compartment of the knee (Point 1) but that normal joint space remains in the lateral compartment.

You might also see osteophytes or spurs—calcified outcroppings at the edges of the tibia, the femur, or the patella. Point 2 on Figure 6-2B shows a spur on the patella. My opinion is that these spurs are the body's attempt to stabilize the joint when it becomes wobbly from cartilage loss. But spurs actually turn into part of the problem because they are rough growths within the joint where there should be only smooth surfaces. Sometimes pieces of these spurs will break off and become loose bodies or

**6-2A**

The front view of an arthritic knee. Point 1 shows the joint space narrowing on the medial side of the knee indicating that the cartilage is virtually gone—there's no longer a cushion for this joint.

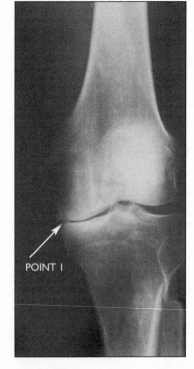

POINT 1

fragments inside the joint. Point 3 shows loose bodies in this knee.

Subchondral cysts show up on X rays as dark, round holes since the bone has been replaced by a fluid-filled cyst. Point 4 shows a subchondral cyst in the patella. To understand how these cysts can form, picture the linoleum on your kitchen floor. If there were a crack in it and you spilled milk on the floor, the milk could seep through to the underlying floorboards and cause them to rot. Similarly, as cartilage cracks in the degenerative process of arthritis, the lubricating fluid in the knee joint can seep through the cartilage to the underlying bone (subchondral bone) and collect there as cysts. These cysts further weaken the cartilage, just as your floor is weakened when termites eat away the floorboards under your kitchen linoleum.

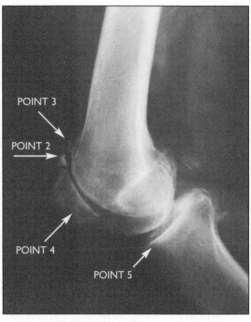

**6-2B**
The side view of an arthritic knee. Point 2 shows a spur on the patella. Point 3 shows a loose body in the joint, and Point 4 shows a subchondral cyst. Point 5 appears where sclerosis is evident in the tibia.

Sclerosis is a hardening of the bone. It's the opposite of osteoporosis. Osteoporosis—fragile bones—shows up on an X ray as washed-out bones, while sclerosis shows up with a denser, whiter-looking bone. Point 5 in Figure 6-2B shows sclerosis in the tibia. As your knee joint becomes arthritic and begins to have problems functioning smoothly, it no longer shares the weight of the body equally on all its surfaces. The weightbearing becomes concentrated in certain spots of the joint and those areas become denser as the body attempts to protect the joint. So the X ray will show more sclerosis—a denser look to the bone in the arthritic knee.

In knees, X rays are considered good overall surveillance: you can look for the four signs of osteoarthritis previously mentioned, you can rule out a bone tumor, and you can make sure there isn't a fracture. Once those things are excluded, if pain persists, an MRI will be needed to help locate the soft tissue source of pain.

When you have an X ray you'll be asked to take a breath and hold it so that you won't inadvertently move. Then you'll hear a buzz and that will be it. There will be no discomfort or sensation.

## MRIs

The MRI is becoming the primary tool for inspecting the knee, which has many internal soft tissue structures. Unlike X rays, the MRI allows you to see both the bones and the soft tissues of the body. This means you can see internal derangement of the knee—meniscal tears, cruciate ligaments tears, and chondromalacia (cartilage thinning) of the patella—three primary things you can't see on an X ray that readily appear on an MRI. You can see swelling, bruising, and inflammation—the same sort of inflammation, for example, that occurs inside the joint at the beginning stages of arthritis. You'll also be able to see fluid inside the joint and inflammation of the joint lining. The MRI image appears in great detail, using different shades of black, white, and gray to bring out actual tissue types, including fat, cartilage, meniscus, tendons, and ligaments.

To understand the difference between an X ray and an MRI, imagine that I have a ten-inch-long candle standing upright in a candle holder and that the wick is filled with calcium. If I take an X ray of that candle, the wax will disappear and the only thing that will show up is the wick running vertically. Now, if I decide I need an MRI of that candle, the image I get of the wick won't be lengthwise, but will instead be a slice right through the candle, and I'll be viewing the wick as if from above. I'll see it sitting like a doughnut hole with the wax as the doughnut all around it. Now I can see the front, back, right, and left side of the wick, not just the vertical length of it. Further, I can see the individual strands that are braided together diagonally to make up the wick, and I can also see any defects in the wax. There will be a series of "slices" showing up in the pictures so we can search for the problem. We will be able to see, for instance, that there's a disruption of the fibers that make up the wick, or that the fibers have been stretched and are no longer oriented correctly.

Then, to identify the location, I look at a localizer reference grid, which will tell me that the first photograph corresponds to the four-inch height level of the candle and the second photograph corresponds to the eight-inch height level. The MRI can take as many slices as are necessary. The radiologist can request ten slices in a ten-inch candle, or he can request thirty. If, for instance, the radiologist is worried that there might be a tear in the meniscus, he can specify thinner cuts, which will provide more pictures and more information.

An X ray tells us what the wick looks like from only one side, top to bottom, but the MRI gives us a three-dimensional look from above at the entire circumference of the wick and the candle—front, back, left, and right—in the multiple places where it has been sliced.

---

**TREAT THE SYMPTOMS, NOT THE FINDINGS**
The findings on the MRI should match the symptoms you have. Even if your MRI results say that you've torn a meniscus, if your symptoms are subsiding, don't rush into surgery. Doctors can operate when the symptoms require it, but not before. Don't let them operate on the findings of a test.

---

Magnetic resonance imaging (MRI) does not use X rays, but magnetism and radio waves. The powerful magnet requires certain precautions that will be explained to you prior to the test.

To have an MRI of your knee, you'll go into a room and see

a large donut-shaped machine. The donut hole is a tube approximately six feet long at its center. The technician will help position you to lie flat on your back on a padded, moveable platform that's about as wide as a stretcher. Your feet will be pointed toward the tube, and you'll have a cushion under your knee. When the test is ready to begin, your body will slide inside the tube until your knee is at the center of the tunnel. Your head and shoulders will remain outside. You'll spend thirty minutes lying motionless in this position while you'll hear rhythmic pounding and whirring sounds. These "closed" MRI systems have great resolution and therefore excellent pictures with great definition. Open MRI scanners have less than one-third the resolution—otherwise, everyone would use them to avoid potential claustrophobia issues. For your knee MRI, your head and shoulders are outside the tube, so that shouldn't be a concern. In the future, open scanners will probably be as good as the closed scanners of today, but for now, the best pictures with the most information come from MRIs done in closed tubes.

In recent years, the bore of MRI tubes has increased in diameter to accommodate those who are large in girth, and the weight limitation for most MRIs has recently been increased from 300 pounds to 350 pounds.

---

**MAKING THE MRI MORE COMFORTABLE**
You might want to shop around for the most comfortable MRI experience. Some units have these amenities: earphones so you can listen to music to drown out the jackhammer sounds of the magnet; a microphone so you can talk to the technician in the control console; a fan that blows air through the tube, giving the comforting sensation of standing in a breeze.

---

## CT SCANS

In the term CT scan or CAT scan, the letters stand for computerized axial tomography. It is a three-dimensional X ray that shows a full picture of the bones from every possible angle. Like the X ray, it shows **only** bone, not the knee's soft tissue structures such as ligaments, tendons, or menisci.

Like the MRI, a CT scan offers "sliced" views of the body as seen from the front, from the side, and from the top. Thus you can see more detail if you have a complicated bone fracture or if your doctor suspects and is looking for osteophytes (spurs), cysts, or sclerosis. All of these are shown perfectly on a CT scan.

For the CT scan, you'll go into a room with a scanner and lie on a narrow platform. The platform slides into a donut-shaped tube that's about two feet deep. Most of your body will be outside the tube, except for the knee portion that is being scanned. The platform will move you through the tube, stopping at specific intervals for each scan. The person taking your scan will be in the control room watching you through a glass window and speaking to you through a microphone. You'll be able to talk to the technician if you're uncomfortable or concerned about anything. Although twenty minutes are usually allotted for the scan, the actual scanning time is approximately forty-five seconds. During that time, you'll need to lie still. You won't feel anything, but you'll hear a whirring sound as the computer moves the X ray machine around your body. Most patients are relatively comfortable during the procedure.

---

**FUTURE MEDICAL RECORDS**

You may eventually have your entire life's medical file, including all the imaging studies and doctors' notes, on a small memory chip embedded in a credit card that you can place in your wallet. If you change doctors, you'll merely swipe your credit card through the new doctor's ATM-like machine and all your data will be there instantly.     —DOUGLAS H. BROWN, M.D.

## Keep Your Own Images

The world of medicine is changing. So are insurance plans, Medicare, and health maintenance organizations (HMOs). Doctors come in and out of your life. The only constant is you. Thus the new digital images that are conveniently kept and carried on a CD are a wonderful way to keep your current X rays, MRIs, and CT scans in your possession and to carry them with you when you visit various doctors.

---

**KEEP YOUR IMAGES AND PHYSICAL HISTORY NOTES**
Keep all your studies on a CD. If you have many studies, your health history library may grow to two or three CDs. If you live in a rural area without a PACS system, ask your doctor for a copy of your X rays and other studies. Keep the films together in the large envelopes they come in, and store them in a cool, dark place. Put them flat on top of everything else in a closet or another location where you won't lose them. Keep a copy of your physical history (see page 93) in the same place and write the date on it. This information will be very useful for comparison over the years to come.

---

Here's an example of how important your prior imaging studies can be. A patient came to me complaining of knee pain. The current MRI showed a loss of circulation to the femur—worrisome, because it could lead to a collapse of the cartilage, then osteoarthritis. But when we looked at his MRI that was taken four years ago in Miami, we saw that the condition had been worse at that time. We could see that his knee was getting better. So instead of planning surgery to improve the circulation to the bone, we took a wait-and-see attitude. Having his old MRI was invaluable.

# 7 THE RIGHT TREATMENT: DOING *YOUR* PART

The fit knee requires daily strengthening and stretching. When your lifestyle is energetic and includes varied activities, your knee is constantly challenged to retain its resiliency and mobility. But when a sore knee slows you down, even forces you to stop your favorite activities altogether, you slide through the Negative Spiral explained on page 37.

By making a commitment to treatment, you can enter the Positive Spiral to knee health shown here.

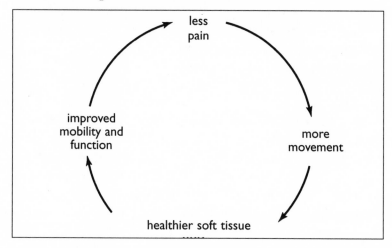

Begin by choosing among these conservative treatments that will allow entry at the point of **less pain**. You can do treatments 1 through 5 on your own. Seek skilled help for treatments 6 through 10. For example, visit a nutritionist for help with planning a healthy diet for weight loss, a physical therapist for therapeutic exercises, a Pilates or yoga instructor for instruction in those disciplines, or an acupuncturist/herbalogist for alternative medicine remedies.

**1. REDUCE HIGH-IMPACT ACTIVITIES.** Reduce the duration of your everyday high-impact activities by **climbing fewer stairs, carrying fewer heavy packages, avoiding standing in long lines, doing less taxing yard work, or walking shorter distances.** And modify your sports life: replace high-impact, abusive activities with the nurturing ones of pool workouts, bicycling, and skiing on a ski machine. (See the Huey-Klapper Activities Point Scale on page 76.)

---

**THE BODY IS INNATELY PROGRAMMED TO HEAL**

When pain is "stuck," or unchanging, it seems the healing process is stuck as well. You need to do something to get "unstuck." All of the treatments described in this chapter can start the process. Once your pain starts shifting location slightly or the symptoms begin changing, the injury is trying to heal. That's what the body is always trying to do.

---

**2. WEAR IMPACT-ABSORBING SHOES.** The harder your shoes, the more impact you are transmitting to all of your weightbearing joints, including your knees. That translates to more trauma to the cartilage and meniscus surfaces. Start wearing highly cushioned athletic shoes made for runners. Such shoes may not be realistic to wear all the time, given the demands and dress codes of your workplace, but wear them whenever you can. Don't wear boots! That extra weight on your foot applies increased pressure directly onto your patella. If you're a boot-lover, take off your boots for one week and feel the difference. Then keep them off except for special occasions.

**3. USE ICE AND HEAT.** Ice is the most under-recognized of all painkillers. It needs no prescription, is easy to apply, is quick to begin working—and it's free. Applying ice to your sore knee reduces blood flow, slows nerve conduction, and elevates your pain threshold. Because it immediately cuts your pain, it decreases your need for pain medication.

Fill a large zip-lock freezer bag with ice cubes. Place a thin cloth or paper towel between the ice bag and your skin. Position the bag on the part of your knee where you feel pain. Leave the ice bag in place for ten to fifteen minutes. When you remove the ice, wrap a dry towel around the cold skin. You will feel the area start to thaw. If your knee hurts in more than one place, move the ice to another sore spot for another ten to fifteen minutes.

For convenience, Ice/Heat by Tru-Fit can be used instead of ice bags. This reusable item consists of a freezable gel pack that fits into an insulated soft fabric encasement. Its stretchy Velcro straps wrap around your knee. The straps stay snugly in place so you can continue your daily activities at home or at work with none of the mess of ice bags. The gel pack can also be heated in the microwave, thus offering contrast ice and heat treatments.

Ice decreases cell metabolism and increases tissue stiffness. Heat increases cell metabolism and decreases tissue stiffness. Both ice and heat decrease pain. Use ice as the **only** treatment for the first forty-eight hours if you have a sudden or acute injury to the knee. If the knee problem is considered chronic, both ice and heat can be used. Apply heat. Follow it immediately with ice. Go back and forth several times: heat, ice, heat, ice, an alternation called "contrast ice and heat." Heat causes vasodilation, an increase of blood supply to the area, then ice brings about vasoconstriction, a decrease in the blood supply. These contrast treatments confuse the body by bombarding it with stimulants that are opposites. The confusion causes an escalated response and a remarkable amount of circulation and healing to the area.

When at home, place your Ice/Heat gel pack in the microwave for one minute to create a hot pack. Cover it in a towel to prevent burning your skin and wrap it around your knee. In fifteen minutes, switch to ten minutes of ice. As the ice treatment begins, you may feel a deepening of the pain, an aching from the cold. Then, as the numbing occurs, virtually all deep pain is gone. When the heat is applied again, the cold tissues go through a "thawing" sensation that most people find pleasurable. Finish your contrast treatment with ten minutes of ice. Hot showers, baths, hot tubs, and cold pools are also appropriate contrast treatments for pain management. In the hot tub, sit in a position that allows the jet stream to flow directly at your knee. And of course you can always use an old-fashioned heating pad in place of your gel pack.

**4. TAKE ANALGESICS OR ANTI-INFLAMMATORIES.** Over-the-counter medications used for joint pain generally fall into two categories: acetaminophens and nonsteroidal anti-inflammatories (Nsaids). Acetaminophen, most commonly found in Tylenol, is an analgesic and antipyretic, which means it relieves pain and lowers fever. Nsaids (aspirin, Advil, or Motrin) relieve pain and reduce fever, plus they also reduce inflammation.

Phone your doctor to ask if you can begin taking these nonprescription analgesics or anti-inflammatories. Your doctor knows the medicines you're already taking. He will tell you how these new drugs interact with your prescription drugs. Commit to using the medicines only for a month or two, knowing you'll soon wean yourself from such pills and depend on the natural drugs your body manufactures when you exercise.

---

**GENE THERAPY**
The day will come, maybe within the next ten years, when surgeons will be able to isolate the gene for osteoarthritis. The child of parents who had OA could have that specific gene clipped or changed before he or she reaches the age of thirty or forty, when the breakdown of the articular cartilage would begin to manifest. Then we will truly have a cure for arthritis.

---

**5. EXERCISE REGULARLY.** Doctors used to believe that exercise caused arthritis as well as the deterioration of crucial cartilage. Now it is known that regular, proper exercise is an excellent way to help the joints stay healthy. While some people with knee problems need to reduce their abusive-type exercises, many others need to break out of being sedentary and begin daily, regular, nurturing exercise. During exercise, some movements "squeeze" the cartilage, pushing out fluids as if from a sponge. Then, when the pressure is released during other phases of movement, nutrient-rich fluids rush back into the cartilage to keep it moist. This pushing out and rushing in of fluids keeps the cartilage from becoming thin, dry, and increasingly susceptible to damage. If you haven't exercised in months or even years, you may decide to seek the help of a professional—an instructor of a low-impact exercise class or a personal trainer with knowledge of knee problems.

**6. EAT HEALTHY FOODS AND MAINTAIN IDEAL BODY WEIGHT.** What you eat will affect your knees, and what you leave out of your diet will do the same. Your body needs a healthy, joint-preserving diet if you want to do everything possible to heal your knees. Read magazines and books about healthy diets or find a nutritionist whose philosophy appeals to you.

Every time you take a step, you load your knees with more than three times your bodyweight, so if you weigh 150 pounds, each knee has to support over 450 pounds with each step! Every pound you gain means more than three pounds of pressure placed on your knee with each step. Conversely, if you were to lose ten pounds, you could eliminate thirty pounds of pressure that your knee must bear.

---

**OBESITY BADLY AFFECTS KNEES**

Researchers have conclusively linked weight gain and obesity to osteoarthritis of the knee. In fact, a large percentage of patients gained weight just before arthritic symptoms appeared. The latest studies performed at the Hospital for Special Surgery in New York City show that obesity (being overweight twenty-five pounds or more) is a key factor in a large percentage of patients needing total knee replacements. Further, obese patients who have this major surgery have a less successful outcome and are also more at risk for complications after surgery. Just as being overweight is one of the worst things you can do to your knees, **reaching or maintaining your ideal body weight is the best thing you can do for your knees.**

---

There's no mystery to losing weight. You have to increase your exercise and cut down on your eating. But with two out of three Americans in the obese category, overweight people now consider themselves just one of the crowd. Changing eating habits can be difficult, especially if other family members are overeaters and unsupportive of dietary cutbacks. Try brushing your teeth immediately after the main course of every meal. It will amaze you how unappealing dessert (or second helpings) will suddenly become.

Most people can't lose weight alone, so get whatever help you need to create an exercise/food-management program with which you're comfortable. Stick with it and really take off some fat. Your knee is at risk, so get serious. Make up your mind: are potato chips, pies, pizza, and hot fudge sundaes more important to you than your knee? As soon as you've chosen your knee, French fries will seem disgusting. Ice cream will lose its appeal. All you will want is a minimal amount of healthy food so you can watch the numbers on the scale go down and down and feel your knee become increasingly capable. **Now is the time to lose weight by dieting and starting a low-impact exercise program.**

7. START PHYSICAL THERAPY. Physical therapists give various treatments, including ultrasound, soft-tissue mobilization, joint mobilization, and therapeutic exercise. Your physical therapist can teach you a home exercise program that will help you safely strengthen the muscles around your knee to provide a cushion to the joint.

### *Ultrasound*

Therapeutic ultrasound mechanically vibrates tissues at an extremely high frequency. This micro-massage raises the tissue's temperature, which improves circulation, resulting in increased cellular metabolism, thus accelerating the healing process. Ultrasound is applied on the skin through a water-based gel. Medications can be added to the gel so the ultrasound drives the medicine through the skin into the underlying tissues. When ultrasound is used in this way, it is called phonophoresis.

> **MODALITIES**
> When doctors or physical therapists speak of using a modality, they are referring to the application of a therapeutic agent—for example, ice, heat, and electrotherapy. They are all modalities, and they help rouse the body's natural healing forces while decreasing pain and swelling. While they can make you feel better, they are strictly an adjunct to the exercises that are the true heart of your program. Modalities can be a temporary solution to pain; improved strength and flexibility are the long-term answer.

### Soft-tissue Mobilization

Muscles, tendons, ligaments, and fascia are soft tissues around your knees. When these tissues are strained, torn, or otherwise damaged, they become restricted, virtually "frozen." A physical therapist can manipulate them with his or her hands to soften the hard, unmoving tissues and help them regain their normal elasticity and movement.

### Joint Mobilization

When a knee joint's mobility is impaired, the structure and function of the knee region begins to change. Adjacent joints (the hip or ankle) begin to move excessively to compensate for the stiff knee. Even cartilage health begins to diminish within the joint. A physical therapist can skillfully apply pressure to move the joint in a desired direction that will help increase motion and normalize knee joint function. Such joint mobilization can improve joint mobility while it decreases muscle spasms and pain.

### Therapeutic Exercise

If regaining the strength and function in your knee were as easy as resuming your former activities, you would be able to rehabilitate yourself. But most people don't know where to draw the line: how much time to exercise, how many repetitions to do, how much strength to exert. A physical therapist is skilled in establishing programs for patients so they can slowly, gradually improve their knee function without overdoing and causing further harm. Chapters 10 and 11 take you inside the world of pool and land physical therapy.

---

**CORTISONE INJECTIONS**

If you have diabetes or a disease in which your immune system is compromised, you should not have a cortisone injection. Further, it is well known in the medical community that injecting cortisone into a joint will damage the surfaces of the vital articular cartilages in that joint. Yes, cortisone is a miraculous anti-inflammatory that knocks out pain and swelling (sometimes temporarily, sometimes forever), but on a cellular level it damages working surfaces of the joint and leaves behind, to linger forever in your joint, the gritty, powdery substance used as a preservative in the cortisone. Repeated injections into a joint literally "spoil" that joint. Doctors know that, but they look at the trade-off. Yes, I've injected cortisone into a knee on exceptional occasions: an actress performing on stage wanted to finish the run of that play; a man wanted to travel to see the birth of a grandchild. In both cases I made sure the patient understood the risk.        —ROBERT KLAPPER, M.D.

---

### 8. CONSIDER MASSAGE THERAPY, ACUPUNCTURE, CHIROPRACTIC, AND HERBAL REMEDIES

#### *Massage Therapy*

By kneading, elongating, and gently manipulating soft tissues beyond their restrictions, the therapist relieves muscle spasms, softens tight and inflamed tendons, increases blood flow, and generally aids in restoring health and function to the knee. When the massage therapist's hands are exerting the pressure to the tissues, you may feel increased pain, but as soon as the pressure is released, your tissues should feel more mobile and less painful.

### Acupuncture

Acupuncture has been used for thousands of years in China, and it has endured for a reason—it obviously helps heal. Acupuncturists use needles to relieve pain and stimulate the body's natural healing systems. While scores of illnesses are treated by acupuncture in Asia, its primary use in the United States has been to relieve chronic pain from such conditions as arthritis, headache, and back pain. Acupuncture for knee problems has shown benefits for those suffering from osteoarthritis and rheumatoid arthritis, knee trauma, and overuse syndromes.

### Chiropractic

Chiropractic comes from the Greek word *chiropraktikos*, which means "effective treatment by hand." Doctors of chiropractic take physical histories, perform a physical exam, and take X rays. They also locate and adjust musculoskeletal areas of the body that function improperly. These adjustments, or manipulations, can free joint and nerve restrictions that cause knee pain, restoring normal function to the muscles, knee joint, and the surrounding nerves. Sometimes a problem in the knee can lead to back pain. In that case, a chiropractor who is skilled in assessing the whole body as well as the spine can work hand in hand with your orthopedic surgeon. Some chiropractors offer the same ultrasound treatments and other modalities offered by physical therapists.

### Herbal Remedies

Ancient Chinese herbal formulas were first introduced over 3,000 years ago. The average practitioner knows about 300 individual herbs that can be combined into thousands of prescriptions. Most formulas consist of two to eighteen different types of herbs that can treat a wide variety of symptoms while stimulating the body's natural healing mechanisms. Anti-inflammatory herbs can be a good alternative to pharmaceutical drugs, especially for those who experience uncomfortable side-effects when taking traditional Nsaids (see page 130). Long-term use of Nsaids can damage the stomach, kidneys, and liver, so herbal remedies might be the best solution for those with chronic conditions, such as osteoarthritis of the knee. Herbs often don't offer the same rapid relief as pharmaceutical drugs, but when properly administered, they can provide a gentle long-term solution to various conditions. Herbs are particularly useful in relieving pain-driven anxiety or the depression that often accompanies chronic physical problems and the loss of favorite activities.

**9. Try Yoga or Pilates.** Yoga offers a series of sustained stretches that can increase your flexibility and strength. Yoga postures are held for several minutes each, and the slow, deep breathing that accompanies these positions reduces muscular tension , anxiety, and pain. As you relax deeply into each sustained stretch, your quadriceps, hamstrings, gastrocs, and knee joints gradually release, giving you more movement.

**Stop any poses that cause undue pain and avoid extreme positions that put unnecessary stress on the knees.**

---

**YOGA**

Choose your yoga class carefully. You'll find a vast array of classes from which to choose, but many of these have diluted yoga's original intent of slow stretches combined with deep breathing and meditation: they've become Westernized "workouts." Search for a class that focuses on lying and sitting stretches, not standing poses and jumping moves. Your intent is to relieve pain, not to stress an already troubled knee joint.

Pilates is an exercise program that aims to develop the body's center, or "core," muscles that create a stable basis for all types of movement. Based on the century-old teachings of Joseph Pilates, this discipline requires a time commitment from both the teacher and the student in order to change and improve the body's postural alignment habits. Like yoga, Pilates professes to be an all-encompassing mind, body, and spiritual exercise. Classes are often one-to-one, which helps maximize the benefits while minimizing risk of injury. Physical therapy clinics often include Pilates as part of their knee rehabilitative exercise regimen.

**10. POOL THERAPY.** Exercising in water is the best of all pain-reducing treatments. It naturally increases circulation, releases endorphins (the body's painkillers), and stimulates the body's healing mechanisms. Your primary treatment for preventing knee surgery, especially if you are overweight, in pain, or have weak muscles, is to begin here, with a pool program.

In Chapter 9 you'll be introduced to the longer, more comprehensive pool program discussed in Chapter 10, which allows you to progress along the Positive Spiral to knee fitness.

# 8 DESIGNING YOUR OWN PROGRAM

*With Tanya Moran-Dougherty, MPT*

Now that you're ready to begin your exercise program, you're probably thinking "Where do I start?" Here are some guidelines to follow for a **safe** progression toward your rehabilitation goals. They are not hard and fast rules—listen to your body. If your pain increases with an exercise, whether that exercise is in the pool or on land, you can perform fewer repetitions, decrease your range of motion (ROM), or skip the exercise altogether. **You** are in charge of your program, which you will design using the pool exercises in Chapters 10 and the land exercises in Chapter 11.

Your body's pain messages are the best guide you have while exercising, so listen carefully. But don't expect your body to tell you the same thing every day, because your pain's location and severity can change. Begin each day's exercise session slowly, monitoring carefully for possible pain. Make adjustments according to what you feel by moving more slowly or more quickly, reaching for more or less range of motion, and adding or subtracting exercises as appropriate.

TREATING AN ACUTE KNEE INJURY

If you sprained your knee but you won't be having surgery, you need to follow a limited program that won't further damage your injury. Ask your doctor if you have a Grade 1, 2, or 3 sprain. Grades 1 and 2 represent partial tears of a ligament. For those, you can follow the postsurgical meniscus program that begins on page 267. If you have a Grade 3 complete tear of a ligament, follow the postsurgical ACL program that begins on page 274.

## GUIDELINES FOR A POOL / LAND REHAB PROGRAM

**Begin by doing the pool exercises three days the first week.** Gently try each exercise in the order presented. If you don't feel increased knee pain, add that exercise to your program. Skip exercises that increase your pain for now. Try to add them to your program again next week. (You'll be amazed how quickly you gain capability in the water!) Do the low-intensity program of deep-water intervals and the lowest number of repetitions of the other exercises. Increase your intensity and reps gradually each week as long as you don't experience increased knee pain and aren't unduly fatigued. If you're tired or sore on any given day, decrease your intensity and reps.

**Skip the Waterpower Workout Exercises 21 to 26 the first few weeks.** These jumping exercises could aggravate your knee, so give your body at least a few weeks to gain strength, flexibility, and overall fitness before trying them. When you first do them, wear a flotation belt. After a few weeks, remove the belt and do the jumps gently again. If any of these exercises increases your knee pain, put your belt back on for another week or two.

**If you're new to exercising, wait until the second week to add two land sessions to your weekly program.** Do the non-weightbearing exercises 1 to 11 on pages 201 to 212. Even if you're experiencing constant pain in your knee, you can perform these gentle ROM and strengthening exercises on a rug, a mat, or a chair at home without harming your knee. Gently try each exercise in the order presented. If you don't feel increased knee pain, add that exercise to your program. Skip exercises that increase your pain for now. Try to add them to your program again next week. Start with one set of ten reps of each exercise.

**As your pain decreases and your strength and mobility improve, increase the number of repetitions.** When ten repetitions is no longer challenging, do two sets of ten reps. When those two sets of ten reps become easy, increase again, this time to three sets of ten. You can gradually increase your workload as long as you don't experience increased knee pain and aren't unduly fatigued. If you're tired or sore on any given day, decrease your reps.

**If you've been exercising four or five times a week in recent months, you can start the first week with three pool *and* two land sessions.** These exercises might seem easy compared to a strenuous, abusive-exercise regimen, but listen to your body during and after every session. Your knee is the weak link in your body chain right now and needs to be respected. If your knee tells you to back off, ice it right away, then skip a day of exercising.

**Perform only land *or* pool exercises on any given day.** You don't want to aggravate your knee by doing too much, so do only one session a day, either pool or land. As you gain strength and capability, you'll add exercises to both your pool and land programs. Soon each of your programs will grow to be quite challenging.

**Allow yourself at least one or two days of rest during**

**the week.** You may be feeling so good that you want to do your exercises every day, but your knee needs time to heal and recover between sessions. If you do the exercises while your muscles are tired or sore you may perform your exercises with improper posture and form, which can lead to further injury to your knee joint and the surrounding tissues. Remember: work + **rest** = improvement. **Plan** the rest days in your program as well as you plan the work days.

**Make the mental connection between pool and land.** Notice that your body is gaining strength and skill in its functional skills (running, walking, lifting, bending, stepping, and squatting) in the pool. Begin visualizing doing those same movements on land, even if you don't yet have enough strength. Soon you'll be doing on land what was so easy in water.

When you can do 20 to 30 step-overs in the pool (Exercise 34, page 194 and 195), it's time for you to begin the land weightbearing Exercises 12 to 15 on pages 212 to 214.

Start with ten reps and when they are no longer challenging, do two sets of ten reps. When those two sets of ten reps become easy, increase again, this time to three sets of ten. Gradually increase your workload each week as long as you don't experience increased knee pain and aren't unduly fatigued. If you're tired or sore on any given day, decrease your reps.

**Continue with the three pool days / two land days combination until you can easily do the following**: 1) POOL: Complete the medium-intensity level of deep-water intervals and do 30 to 50 repetitions of the other pool exercises; 2) LAND: Safely perform all the weightbearing exercises. **Then you're ready to switch to three days of land exercise and two days of pool.** Although you may enjoy the pool work, you need to function well on land, so now you should devote time to mastering functional exercises 16 to 21 (see pages 214 to 218). Start with ten reps of each exercise. When they are no longer challenging, do two sets of ten reps. When two sets of ten reps become easy, increase to three sets of ten. If your knee is sore on any given day, decrease your reps.

**If your knee is swollen or sore after a workout, but you "sleep it off" overnight, keep going with your program.** However, if you experience pain or increased swelling that does not resolve within twenty-four hours, stop. Ice your knee and wait a day or two before resuming a milder version of your previous exercise sessions.

---

**ICE YOUR KNEE AFTER EVERY POOL AND LAND SESSION**
Ice is nature's best anti-inflammatory. Apply ice to your knee after every exercise session, for ten to fifteen minutes. If you don't have an ice pack, a large bag of frozen peas works well. In fact, frozen peas offer more uniform cooling than large ice cubes in a plastic bag. To prevent an ice burn, place the ice inside a towel or pillowcase rather than directly on your skin. (See pages 129 to 130 for more details about icing your knee.)

---

## GUIDELINES FOR A LAND-ONLY REHAB PROGRAM

While the ideal is to do the combined pool and land exercise program described, you may not have access to a pool. Or you may be sensitive to chlorine or afraid of the water. If you can make the effort to find a pool or overcome your concerns, your knee may begin moving sooner and with less pain than if you do land exercises **only**. However, if you must have a program you can do at home, here's how to design your land-only program.

**Try to begin with three exercise sessions the first week.** This is the ideal, but if knee pain has limited your ability to exercise over the past few months, you may need to start with one or two sessions the first week. Listen to your knee as well as the rest of your body. If you're very deconditioned or have trouble doing your normal activities of daily living, do only one to two land exercise sessions a week until the exercises become easy. Then progress to three sessions per week.

**Begin with the non-weightbearing Exercises 1 to 11 only.** For the first few weeks, perform only one set of ten reps. Let pain be your guide. If an exercise increases your pain, decrease your ROM or skip the exercise altogether. If you're performing the exercises properly in your painfree ROM, you should experience very little discomfort doing one set of ten reps.

**When you can stand on your affected leg for at least five seconds without pain or instability, you're ready to begin adding the weightbearing Exercises 12 to 15.** If you're doing the land sessions three times a week, you'll probably be able to do this by the time you've completed two weeks (six sessions). If you don't feel pain when standing on one leg but balance is a problem, do the weightbearing exercises holding a table, counter, or chair until your balance improves. Complete one set of ten reps of Exercises 1 to 11, then add one set of ten reps of Exercises 12 to 15. When that increased workload becomes easy, do two sets of ten reps of Exercises 1 to 15.

**When you can do two sets of ten reps of Exercises 1 to 15 three times a week, you're ready to add the functional Exercises 16 to 21.** You'll probably reach this stage three to four weeks into your rehab program. Try each exercise in the order presented. If you can do an exercise without increased pain, add it to your program. If an exercise increases your knee pain, limit your ROM, hold onto a counter or chair, or skip it for now. You can try the exercises you skipped again next week. After completing two sets of ten reps of Exercises 1 to 15, add one set of ten reps of each of the functional exercises to your program. When your growing program is no longer challenging, do two sets of ten reps of Exercises 1 to 21. When that workload becomes easy, increase to three sets of ten reps.

**Thera-Band exercises add resistance to advanced programs.** Once you've mastered Exercises 1 to 21, add a Thera-Band to your routine for more resistance, as in Exercises 22 to 25. If you experience symptoms after increasing your resistance, use either an easier-strength Thera-Band (see pages 218 and 219) or do the exercises without a band for a few sessions.

Refer back to this chapter many times as you learn the pool and land exercises and use them to design your own personalized knee fitness program. With them, you may be able to prevent, or at least delay for many years, a knee surgery.

# 9 BEFORE YOU RETURN TO THE POOL

When a knee becomes disabled, you can't move well, at least not on land. But in water you're able to move more naturally. Water's magic lies in its buoyant support for the body, its resistance to bodily movement, the pressure it exerts on a submerged body, its ability to reduce pain, and its relaxing and refreshing feel.

Buoyancy is the upward thrust exerted by water on a body that is totally or partially immersed in it. It lifts the body and provides a feeling of weightlessness. If you stand in waist-deep water, fifty percent of your body weight is supported by the water. If you move to chest-deep water, seventy-five percent of your body weight is lifted from your weightbearing joints. In neck-deep water, ninety percent of your body's weight is eliminated. And if you put on a flotation belt and move to deep water, you are virtually weightless. By thus neutralizing gravity's downward force on your knees, you are able to exercise in greater comfort and perform movements that are impossible on land.

The resistance the water supplies to the body during movement is considered the workload, just as a stack of weights in the gym is the workload during a weight-training session. Water offers isokinetic resistance, meaning that it matches the resistance you give it. As hard as you push, it pushes back with equal force. This is a safe and efficient way to strengthen even the sorest knee, because you'll never generate more resistance than you can handle. The resistance always equals the force applied.

The amount of resistance the body encounters in water is directly proportional to the speed of the movement. For example, if you move your leg at a slow speed through the water, you feel a gentle resistance. Then, if you move your leg exactly twice as fast through the water, you will encounter exactly twice the resistance. The water automatically adapts to your demands and becomes an instantly-variable training gym. You can do less work or more, move slower or faster, on any given exercise, depending upon what you feel or need.

The hydrostatic pressure exerted by the water on the submerged surfaces of the body is proportional to the depth of submersion. Therefore, the deeper you are in the water, the greater the hydrostatic pressure. Think of the water as working on your entire body, just as a support stocking works to keep feet, ankles, and calves from swelling. Hydrostatic pressure helps venous blood return to the heart, and it relieves swelling, especially in the arms and legs. As you move, the massaging effect of the water on your body helps loosen and lengthen tight muscles while the hydrostatic pressure helps flush out waste products, such as lactic acid, from tired tissues.

The sensation of water on your skin acts as a counterirritant to reduce your pain. Because nerve impulses stimulated by water on your skin are faster than those stimulated by pain, the skin impulses literally beat the pain impulses to the brain for recognition. The end result is reduced pain.

Exercising in water promotes relaxation. The water encourages you to perform gentle, rhythmic motions, which can reduce muscular tension and improve limited range of movement. Further, the mental and emotional stress that come with pain and impaired physical capability is immediately reduced when you begin movement in water. You perceive less pain and feel more capable, so your body and mind start to relax.

---

**REGAINING MOTION**

Hydrostatic pressure may have another interesting benefit. It may be that the stimulus of the water against your skin provides a valuable communication between the brain, the muscles, and the joint. If your knee's natural monitoring mechanisms—its proprioceptors—have been removed or damaged due to surgery or injury, you may learn to estimate your knee's angle of bend by using information supplied by the sensation of the water against your skin. That extra communication link can help guide you safely through your pool program as you regain motion that has left your movement vocabulary.

---

## THE EQUIPMENT YOU'LL NEED

To do the ten-minute pool program in Chapter 1, you needed no equipment, only a bathing suit. But for the full program in Chapter 10, you'll need a flotation belt so that you can be completely non-weightbearing in deep water. As your strength improves you may add other items for challenge and variety. (A list of all equipment can be found in the Appendix that starts on page 296.)

YOUR SUIT. Men should choose a comfortable pair of trunks. Be sure they have a tie string to make them snug around the waist so they will stay up when you jump or bounce. Women should wear one-piece workout suits, not sun-bathing fashion suits or bikinis. You will be performing a variety of exercises and won't want to be distracted from your form and technique by having to hold your suit in place.

**FLOTATION BELTS.** Flotation belts support the body in deep water, allowing for full range of motion of both arms and both legs in all body positions, from vertical to horizontal. Every flotation belt has its advantages, including plush or rough feel, more or less buoyancy, bright or dull colors. (These belts are identified in the pool photos in Chapter 10.) Each one has its unique properties that should be considered before making a selection. Choosing the wrong belt can make you uncomfortable in the pool, either because it doesn't hold you high enough in the water or because it presses on your ribcage, your chest, or your thighs. Short people should choose a belt that is narrow at the front: the Wet Sweat belt, the Wave belt, or the AquaJogger. Tall people have more room between their rib cages and hips and therefore can comfortably wear the wider H.A.N. belt or Hydro-Tone belt. Athletes, dancers, and others who are muscular will need the most possible buoyancy, which is supplied by the Wet Sweat, H.A.N., and Hydro-Tone belts. People who are "sinkers"—those with little body fat and dense musculature—need to wear two belts, one on top of the other. While this may feel restrictive and even uncomfortable at first, you need to be high enough in the water that you don't lift your chin, altering your head position, which affects your entire body's position. The best two-belt combination for the most comfort is either the H.A.N. belt or the Hydro-Tone belt closest to the body, with the Wave belt on top. The H.A.N. belt is best for those with lower back pain because it acts like an orthopedic corset. It is, however, harder to strap around yourself. The Hydro-Tone belt, by contrast, is easily set to your own waist size and is attached with quick-release buckles. The Wet Sweat and Wave belts are easiest to pack for travel because they're narrow and they dry quickly. (See the following table for a summary of the belts' various features.)

| Flotation Belt Comparison | | | | | |
|---|---|---|---|---|---|
| | BOUYANCY LEVEL | NARROW FRONT | WIDE FRONT | EASY ON/OFF | TRAVEL EASE |
| 2-belt combo | highest | | ✓ | | hard |
| Hydro-Tone | high | | ✓ | ✓ | easy |
| H.A.N. | high | | ✓ | | hardest |
| Wet Sweat | medium | ✓ | | ✓ | easiest |
| AquaJogger | medium | ✓ | | ✓ | easy |
| Wave | low | ✓ | | ✓ | easiest |

RESISTANCE EQUIPMENT. All of the following resistance pieces force the body to move larger volumes of water with each exercise. In effect, this is the equivalent of lifting more weight in the gym, and is very effective strength training. Resistance equipment should not be added to your program until your knee has been painfree for several weeks. At that time, you can add either a flotation ankle cuff or a resistance boot. The ankle cuffs help you bend and straighten a stiff knee while the boot offers maximum resistance to your muscles, increasing your strength.

OTHER HELPFUL EQUIPMENT. Additional equipment can add comfort and stability to your pool session. As your pool program becomes a way of life, you may want to invest in some of these pieces as well.

Comfortable pool shoes protect your feet and provide traction and safety as they reduce the possibility of slipping and falling. If you tend to blister easily or if your pool bottom is slippery, wear pool shoes. If you have diabetes, rheumatoid arthritis, or have had a joint implant, you should **always** wear shoes, not only in the pool but going to and from the locker rooms as well.

A tether fits snugly over your flotation device and attaches from your waist to the side of the pool. (See photo

10-4 on page 163.) This tether provides stability and significantly improves your posture when deep-water running and walking. In shallow water, the tether lets you run at top speed without slipping or moving around the pool. In a large, public pool, you can make your location known to all swimmers by tethering yourself in one spot and staying there while you do your deep-water exercises.

CLOTHING TO KEEP YOU WARM. When you first begin the knee pool program, you may be moving quite slowly. If your pool temperature is the standard 82 to 84 degrees, you'll probably find yourself getting cold and starting to shiver within twenty minutes. In order to be comfortable in cool water, consider investing in a surfer-like piece of attire that is specifically designed to keep you warm. Pullover Thermo X shirts are fleece-lined, stretch, and offer protection from the sun's UV rays as well as a luxurious layer of warmth against cool water. They come in either long-sleeved or short-sleeved styles. A Neoprene, short-sleeve, zip-up shirt is even warmer. (All attire is listed in the Appendix.)

## THE POOL

You may have a pool in your backyard or at your gym. Or you may have to search to find one that will provide you with the depth of water you need and the appropriate temperature. This search is a worthy effort, for pool therapy may save you thousands of dollars in other kinds of treatment.

Nowadays nearly every community has a pool that can be used for a small fee. Your local college, YMCA, YWCA, YMHA, and community recreation department are your best bets for finding inexpensive access to pools. Health club membership fees can be expensive, but they usually have many amenities, including a sauna, steam room, or jacuzzi. Local hotels may offer pool memberships to the neighborhood.

The pool you use for knee rehabilitation should have a shallow end with chest-deep water for your specific height. For example, if you are 5'3", chest-deep water is approximately 3'9". If you are 6' tall, chest-deep water is closer to 4'6". You ideally want to have a relatively flat or unslanted pool bottom so you can walk across the pool at that correct depth. Additionally, you need water that is deep enough so your feet won't touch the bottom of the pool. For most people, this means you need water at least six feet deep.

When you first begin your program, you might be moving quite slowly, so water temperatures of 89 to 93 degrees will be most comfortable for you. Few pools are this warm —mostly those that are dedicated to water therapy. As you progress and begin moving more strenuously, you'll feel comfortable in water that is 85 to 88 degrees. Again, few pools are kept this warm. Public pools normally cater to lap swimmers who prefer cool water around 80 degrees. Multiuse pools that have a large number of water exercisers often compromise, keeping the water at 82 to 85 degrees. It may be hard to find a pool of the perfect depth and ideal water temperature, so if you have to decide between the two, choose a pool that has the proper depth of water for you, even if the water is cooler than you'd like. You can always make yourself warmer with additional protective clothing, previously mentioned.

Check your potential pool's schedule. Make sure there is a recreational swim time during which you can use the pool without interference from lap-swimmers, children, or divers. Ideally the pool you choose for your water training should be no more than ten to fifteen minutes from your home or your workplace. The locker room should be clean and inviting. If your "home" pool is easily accessible, and if you are comfortable in its surroundings, you'll use it more often than if it is unattractive or a long drive away.

And find a back-up pool for emergency use. You'd hate to see an unexpected Closed sign on your main pool and have to miss your therapy for a week just because you hadn't located an alternate pool.

## IF YOU BUILD YOUR OWN POOL

Many people eventually decide to build their own backyard pools to meet their specific needs. Should you make the decision to build your own pool, consider these ideas in your planning:

- Think of the annual weather pattern in your area. If you don't have at least four to five months of weather good enough for outdoor pool exercise, think again. A small indoor tank or health club membership might be more appropriate for you.
- Consider the amount of sunlight you have in your backyard. You don't want a pool that's in the shade all day, but one that's mostly in the sun.
- Pay attention to the surrounding trees and think of how much wind you have and from which prevailing direction. Consider the leaves, flowers, or other droppings that will fall into your pool, depending on where you place it.
- Ask friends and business associates for names of reputable pool builders. Interview at least three builders and get names of pool owners in your area whom you can visit to see their pools and ask questions about the building process.
- Plan approximately equal amounts of shallow and deep water in your pool. Without the appropriate depth of shallow water, you can't do gait training and knee exercises well. Without deep water, you're not able to do non-weightbearing exercises.

- If your pool will be relatively small, you may need to ask the builder to create a flat, not slanted, shallow end, so that you can do your gait training in chest-deep water. Measure from the ground to the middle of your chest to see exactly how deep your shallow water should be. If two or more people of differing heights intend to use the pool, you may have to compromise by selecting an average chest-height depth.
  - You also need water that is deep enough so your feet won't touch the bottom of the pool. For most people, this means you need water at least six feet deep. When building small pools, you may have to ask your city for a variance to the standard pool-building permit so that you can have one unvarying depth in the shallow end, then let the bottom make a 90-degree drop off into the deep end.
- Place bars to hold during stretching exercises in both the deep and shallow ends, facing away from the dominant direction of the sun.
- Plan your stairs into the pool to have a shorter rise than normal stairs. For instance, make four easy steps down into the pool rather than three steeper steps.
- Add two railings going down your stairs so you can walk between them. You can hold one bar in each hand and comfortably lower yourself down the steps. If you build a spa, add another set of railings to help you in and out.
- Instead of stairs, consider a ramp. Ramps provide a slanted walkway into the pool for easier access.
- Design a square or rectangular pool so an electric cover can easily be installed to keep your pool warm a few extra months each year or even year-round. Odd-shaped pools can make adding a pool cover virtually impossible. If you add a spa, place it inside the pool perimeter so it, too, can be covered when not in use.

- Consider solar heating, which in the long-run will cut down on your gas bill for heating the water.

One final consideration before you begin your pool program. Keep in mind that you feel less pain in the water than on land, and because you may not feel the pain of a new movement until the next day, err on the side of caution as you begin your pool recovery.

# 10 A POOL EXERCISE PROGRAM FOR KNEES

**If you've recently had knee surgery, turn to Chapter 14 for help in pacing yourself correctly through this program. Find your specific surgery type and follow its guidelines.**
To restore the function of your knee, you must increase the strength of the muscles surrounding the knee and must regain weightbearing capability by safely and gradually increasing the amount of impact your knee can tolerate. As you begin to accomplish both of these goals in the pool, you'll gain at least one wonderful, perhaps unexpected, benefit. Your entire body will become stronger and more flexible; you'll develop better cardiovascular capacity and move more efficiently—you'll simply feel better.

If you're comfortable in deep water, put on your flotation belt and begin with Exercise 1. (See pages 150 and 151 for guidance in selecting a flotation device.) Your program contains exercises in both deep and shallow water. If you're a nonswimmer or afraid of the water, move straight to Exercise 8 in shallow water. Over time you will gain confidence in the water and can add Exercises 1 to 7 to your program by holding the side of the pool as you do them. You'll want to add those deep-water exercises in order to be non-weight-bearing and therefore help your sore knee the most.

If you need help remembering your exercises, photocopy the pictures from this chapter, then cut and paste them onto the front and back of one sheet. Laminate the sheet to take to the pool with you. Place it poolside and follow the order of the exercises.

## DEEP EXERCISES

---

**START DEEP-WATER WALKING SLOWLY**
Begin Exercise 1, Deep-water walking, slowly. A lot of force is required to swing straight legs through the water's resistance. It is possible to strain your hip flexor muscles from working too fast too soon, so increase your speed very gradually over several weeks.

---

### EXERCISE 1. DEEP WATER WALKING—BASIC WALK, POWER WALK, SPEED WALK

Start in an upright position, with no forward or backward lean. Hold your right arm and your left leg forward at the same time to establish your "opposition" position. Then begin an exaggerated walking motion, one in which the knees **never** bend. Swing your arms and legs forward and backward—right arm with left leg and left arm with right leg—in a smooth, flowing motion (see photo 10-1A). If you encounter knee pain while doing this, try "locking" your knees to keep the joint stable. If a locked knee increases your pain, try doing these walking exercises with a slightly bent knee.

**Power Walk.** Turn your hands so the palms face backward and they're wide, like paddles. This creates increased resistance for your shoulders, chest, and back. In order to create more work for your calf muscles, flex the foot on the

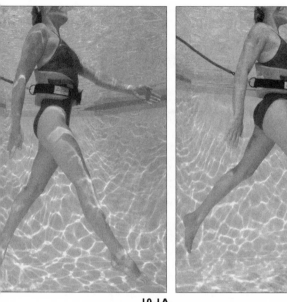
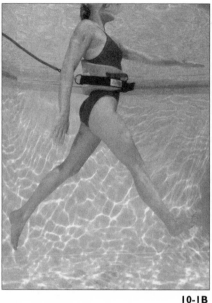
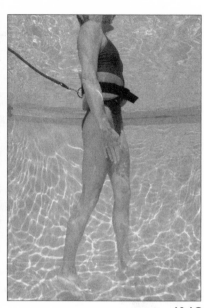

10-1A        10-1B        10-1C

10-1A: Basic walk; 10-1B: Power walk; and 10-1C Speed walk
(all shown with Wet Sweat belt and tether).

leg that swings forward and point the foot on the leg that
swings backward. One foot is flexing and one foot is pointing on each step (see photo 10-1B).

**Speed Walk.** Turn your hands with the thumbs forward so
they "slice" through the water. Your elbows and knees
remain straight throughout the exercise. Tighten your
abdominal muscles and your gluteal (buttocks) muscles to
create a solid torso from which to rapidly swing your arms
and legs. Lift your toes so your feet are flat, as if you were
standing on land. This helps you keep your knees from bending. Narrow the forward and backward range of motion of
your legs so they swing forward and backward less than a
foot or so (see photo 10-1C). Now quicken your steps as you
carefully hold your opposition position. If your shoulders
begin to wobble, you've lost the opposition. Slow down and
start again, gradually building the speed.

## EXERCISE 2. FLIES

Lean slightly backward on this exercise until you find the balance point and it becomes easy for you to do. Start with your arms and legs together as in photo 10-2A. Open your arms and legs out to the position shown in photo 10-2B. Return to the starting position. Keep your hands face-down in a position of minimum resistance against the water. Don't pull your hands downward toward your hips, because that will cause you to bob too high and low in the water. If you find yourself drifting backward toward the side of the pool, turn your palms outward each time you open your arms to help keep yourself in place.

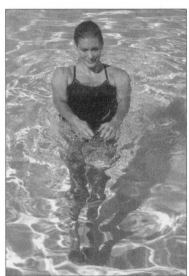

**10-2A** Flies

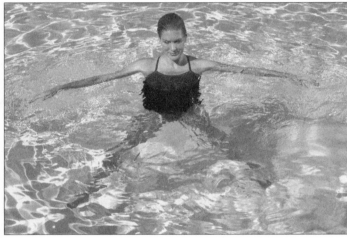

**10-2B**
(HAN belt shown)

## EXERCISE 3. DEEP-WATER RUNNING

If deep-water running increases you knee pain, skip it and you can run later in the program in chest-deep water. Those people with severe osteoarthritis or patellofemoral tracking problems are most likely to experience discomfort from deep-water running.

Run in an upright position using the exact motion of good running form on land. Lift each knee, then push each foot straight down behind you, following the path of the arrow in photo 10-3. Start slowly with minimal bending of your knees at first. If your knee tolerates this, then you can try increasing your speed and lifting your knees up to 90 degrees. Focus your eyes on a point straight ahead that will help you keep your head level and unmoving. Keep your chest erect and your shoulders relaxed and down. Pull your arms forward and backward with no lateral movement. Relax your hands and pull your elbows straight back, each in its turn. Don't lean too far forward or you'll be dog paddling. Don't lean too far back, or you'll start kicking into a bicycling motion.

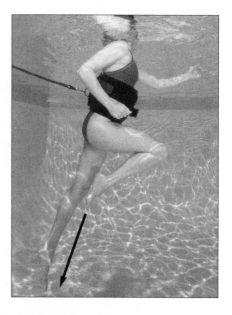

**10-3**
Deep-water running (HAN belt and tether shown)

### STRAIGHT-LEG PROGRAM

If your knee hurts too much to bend, start with this straight-leg program, which helps strengthen your whole body even without bending your knee. A week later, gently try the other exercises again to see if you can add any of them to your program. If not, keep trying each week until you're able to add the other exercises.

Exercise 1. Deep-water walking

Exercise 2. Flies

Exercise 4. Intervals using only Exercises 1 and 2

Exercise 8. Flutter kick—front and back

Exercise 10. Straight-leg deep kick

Exercise 11. Scissors

Exercise 12. Shallow-water walking

Exercise 16. Hamstring stretch

Exercise 20. Gastroc stretch

Exercise 28. Lateral leg raises

Exercise 29. Standing leg swings

Exercise 33. Heel/toe raises

## Deep-Water Interval Training

You will use the skills you learned in Exercises 1 to 3 to create a powerful cardiovascular series. If running hurts your knee, you'll use only Exercises 1 and 2.

Interval training involves performing a challenging work period, then resting, then working again. Basic walk, power walk, and running can all be used as work periods when performed quickly, or they can be used as recovery periods when done slowly. Speed walk is always a work period. Flies, always done slowly, are used as recovery periods. If your knee is quite sore when you first begin this program, you may not be challenging your cardiovascular system and may not require much of a rest period. However, as your knee heals and can withstand more force, you'll be able to increase the effort and speed of these intervals and raise your working heart rate to whatever level you desire.

All of these intervals begin slowly and gradually increase in intensity. **If you feel an increase of pain in your knee at any time, slow down.** If you have any concerns for your heart, discuss this program with your physician before beginning, and monitor your heart rate where suggested.

### EXERCISE 4. INTERVALS

Begin with the low-intensity program the first day. You won't know until the next day if your knee or your muscles are going to be sore or if you will become overly fatigued, so even if the intervals seem too easy, don't move up to the medium-intensity program until the next session. If you begin the medium-intensity program on your second day in the pool, and they again seem too easy, follow the same rule as before: don't move up to the high-intensity program until the next session. Wait to see how your body responds after exercise. If the low- or medium-intensity program suits you well, stick with it for several weeks before attempting to move to a higher-intensity. It's better to make slower, steadier progress than to hurt your knee trying to do work you're not ready for. Such a mistake will force you backward for a week, or even two, to recover. It may have taken many months or even years to develop your knee condition; accept the fact that it may take just as long to help correct it.

Use a Waterpower Workout tether (see Appendix) to maintain good form and position in the pool. Attach it to a ladder, a lane divider, or a piece of lawn furniture (see photo 10-4).

### LOW INTENSITY

Basic walk or power walk (slow), one minute

Flies, one minute

Water run (slow, if no increase in knee pain), one minute

Basic walk or power walk (slow), two minutes

Flies, two minutes

Water run (slow, if no increase in knee pain), two minutes

(Heart-rate check)

Repeat this sequence per your tolerance.

If you had to delete running, replace those minutes with power walk.

Total time: 9:00, or 18:00 if repeated.

### MEDIUM INTENSITY

Basic walk or power walk (slow), two minutes

Flies, two minutes

Water run (slow, if no increase in knee pain), two minutes

Basic walk or power walk (moderate), one minute

Speed walk (fast), one minute

Water run (slow, or moderate, as long as no increase in knee pain), two minutes

Basic walk or power walk (moderate), two minutes

Speed walk (fast), one minute

(Heart-rate check)

If you had to delete running, replace those minutes with power walk.

Repeat this sequence if your stamina and your knee allow.

Total time: 12:00, or 24:00 if repeated.

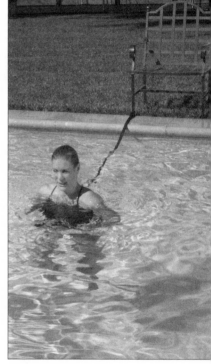

**10-4**
Intervals, tethered to a patio chair

Even if your fitness level can handle a high-intensity series of intervals, you must remember to defer to your knee. If working fast and hard against the water resistance increases the pain in your knee, **slow down**. If walking is easier on your knee than running, do your fastest, hardest intervals in power walk and speed walk modes and your slower and more moderate intervals while running. Skip running altogether if it causes too much pain.

### HIGH INTENSITY

Power walk (easy) one minute

Power walk (moderate) one minute

Flies, one minute

Water run (easy, if no increase in knee pain), one minute

Water run (moderate, if no increase in knee pain), one minute

Power walk (hard), two minutes

(Heart-rate check)

Flies, one minute

Speed walk (fast), one minute

Power walk (hard), one minute

Flies, one minute

Water run two x one-minute buildup (if no increase in knee pain), increasing pace every fifteen seconds to create a four-speed interval: slow, medium, fast, sprint. No rest. Immediately repeat one-minute buildup: slow, medium, fast, sprint.

(Heart-rate check)

Power walk, (hard), one minute. No rest.

Speed walk, (fast), one minute. No rest.

Power walk, (hard), one minute

(Heart-rate check)

Repeat this sequence if your stamina and your knee allow. Eliminate running if your knee is getting sore and work hard on the walking intervals.

Total time: 15:00 to 30:00

Gradually increase the difficulty of your intervals over the next weeks and months. Use what you've learned about interval training from the examples to create your own personalized interval session that lasts fifteen to twenty-five minutes. Vary your session from day to day to avoid losing interest.

## Deep-Waterpower Exercises

If these exercises are hard for you to do as shown, or if you're a nonswimmer, you can hold onto the gutter, a ladder, or the side of the pool. Start all exercises slowly. Then, if you feel no knee pain, gradually increase your speed. If you did the low-intensity intervals, start with ten repetitions of each; moderate-intensity intervals, do twenty reps; and high-intensity intervals, do thirty reps.

### EXERCISE 5. SIT KICKS

Assume a chair-sitting position as shown in photo 10-5. Move your hands gently from side to side in front of you for balance. Gently kick your left foot forward and simultaneously pull the right heel toward your buttocks. Continue alternating one foot forward and the other foot backward. Each right-left kick is one repetition.

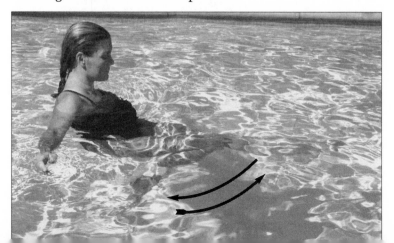

**10-5**
Sit kicks (HAN belt shown)

## EXERCISE 6. HEEL LIFTS

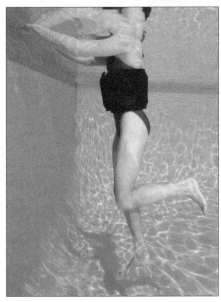

Continue floating and moving your hands gently from side to side for balance, or hold onto the edge of the pool as shown in photo 10-6. Lift your left heel toward your buttocks, then switch feet. One heel lifts while the other foot simultaneously pushes back toward the pool bottom. Each right-left kick is one rep.

## EXERCISE 7. ABDOMINALS

Lean back to find a balanced position in the water as in photo 10-7A. Keep your legs together as you pull both knees toward your chest and your hands toward your knees (see photo 10-7B). Then push your arms and legs back to the starting position. Turn your palms outward on the backward push to maintain your position in the pool.

**10-6** Heel Lifts (HAN belt shown)

**10-7A** Abdominals (Wet Sweat belt shown)

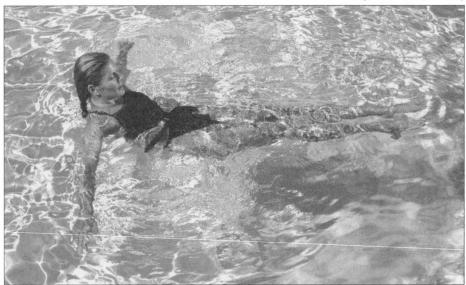

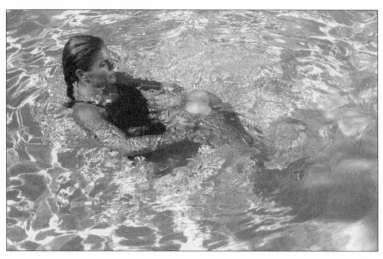

10-7B

*Variation:* If you have trouble balancing on this exercise, you can do it in a vertical position as shown in photos 10-7C and 10-7D. You'll have to focus on performing a powerful isometric contraction of the abdominals each time you lift the knees in order to gain mid-body strength. Otherwise, the exercise uses only the hip flexor muscles, not the abdominals as intended.

10-7D

10-7C

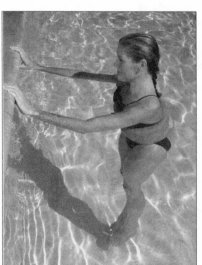

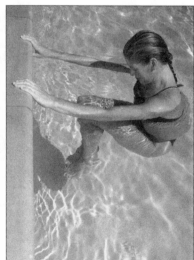

## Shallow or Deep

You can do Kick Training Exercises 8 to 11 in deep water or in shallow water, with a flotation belt or without one. If you skipped Exercises 1 to 7 because you didn't want to work in deep water, begin here in shallow water without a flotation belt. If you've already done Exercises 1 to 7, the most logical progression is to keep your flotation belt on and stay in deep water for Exercises 8 to 11 in this section.

## Kick Training

Find the most comfortable position for your arms on the gutter or lip of the pool. That position may change from exercise to exercise. Experiment to keep your shoulders comfortable. You may prefer to do all these kicks on the steps of your pool. If you feel knee pain, slow your kicking movements or drop your feet below the surface of the water. If you still feel pain, stop that exercise but gently try the next. Re-try the kick that caused pain each time you return to the pool. You'll soon be able to do it.

### EXERCISE 8. FLUTTER KICK—FRONT/BACK

Brace yourself, facing the side of the pool, with your legs floating behind you toward the surface of the water (see photo 10-8A). Hold the pool lip with one hand and place the other hand a foot lower to provide maximum leverage for keeping your legs afloat. Begin tiny flutter kicks with straight legs. If you do your flutter kicks on a step or ledge, keep your elbows bent so your shoulders are under the water and you don't strain your back. Do thirty to sixty left-right repetitions.

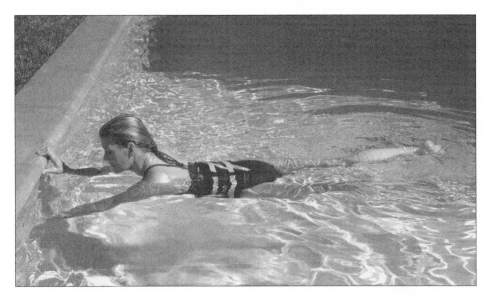

Now turn over so your back is to the wall and brace yourself with your arms on the edge of the pool. Lift your hips and legs and begin shallow flutter kicks with straight legs (see photo 10-8B). If you do your kicking series on a step or ledge, stay low in the water. Do thirty to sixty right-left repetitions.

**10-8A** Front flutter kick (Hydro-Tone belt shown)

**10-8B** Back flutter kick (Hydro-Tone belt shown)

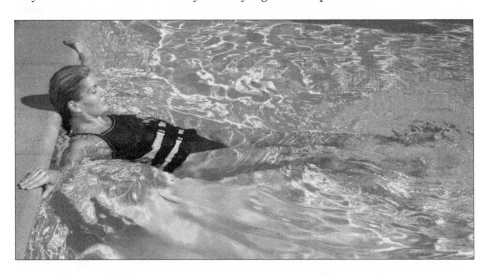

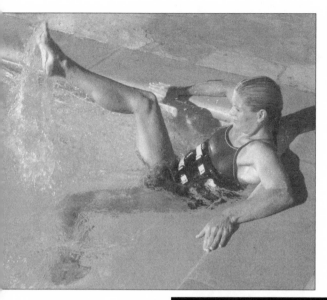

## EXERCISE 9. BICYCLE KICK

Remain braced at the side of the pool or move into a corner for improved shoulder comfort, as shown in photo 10-9. Bend your knees to begin kicking in a bicycling movement. Do twenty to fifty right-left repetitions.

**10-9** Bicycle kick
(Hydro-Tone belt shown)

## EXERCISE 10. STRAIGHT-LEG DEEP KICK

Keep both legs straight throughout this exercise. Lift your left leg to the water's surface while you push the right leg toward the pool bottom (see photo 10-10). Now push the left leg down and lift the right leg toward the surface. Keep exchanging the leg positions until you have completed twenty to thirty right-left reps.

**10-10** Straight-leg deep kick
(Hydro-Tone belt shown)

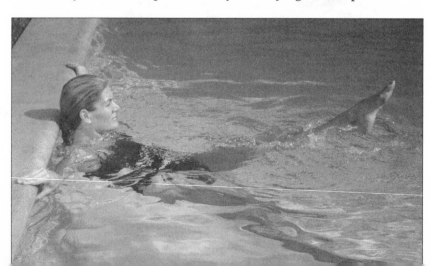

## EXERCISE 11. SCISSORS

If you're wearing a belt, let your body continue to float slightly away from the pool wall. If you're not wearing a belt, push your lower back against the side of the pool and brace yourself against the pool wall. Open your legs wide (see photo 10-11A). Then with a scissors motion, cross one leg over the top of the other, as shown in photo 10-11B. Continue crossing and opening them, alternating the top leg. Use as much force in opening the legs as you use in crossing them. Make sure your knees point upward, not outward. Do twenty to thirty openings and crossings.

**10-11A** Scissors
(Hydro-Tone belt shown)

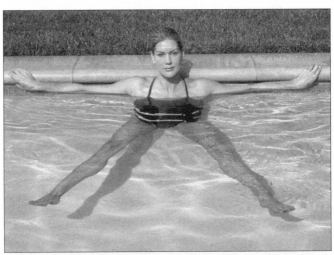

**10-11B**

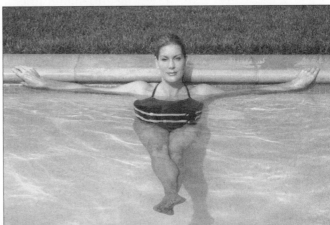

## SHALLOW PROGRAM

Those who have been in deep water should now go to the shallow end of the pool and remove their flotation belts for the rest of the program.

### Gait Training

You may have damaged your knee in a sudden injury or it may have taken months or years for your knee condition to develop. Either way, you have probably found that your normal walking pattern has become irregular due to pain or limitation of the knee's movement. If walking on land causes you knee pain or discomfort, you'll find it a welcome relief to have most of your weight lifted off your knee joint while you walk in the water. In chest-deep water, you can walk relatively pain-free and at the same time refine or relearn the correct biomechanics of walking.

Water shoes can protect your feet and provide traction and safety as they reduce the possibility of slipping and falling. If you have diabetes, rheumatoid arthritis, or if you've had knee or hip implant surgery, you should **always** wear shoes, not only in the pool but going to and from the pool as well. You want to take every precaution not to step on anything and get an infection.

Walk back and forth across the width of a pool if possible so you will have the same depth of water and same amount of water resistance throughout the exercise. You can still get the job done if you must walk the length of the pool in one lane; however, you will find yourself constantly adjusting to a changing amount of buoyancy and resistance if the depth of the water is different at various sections of the pool.

If you feel pain in your knee when you step on it, try these **basic modifications:**
1) move to slightly deeper water,
2) take smaller steps,
3) strap on your flotation belt.

Before performing Exercises 12 to 14, spend a moment trying to visualize yourself walking tall, straight, and without any limp or deviation in your gait. Picture your feet and knees always facing forward and your hips and shoulders always level, never rocking up and down or from side to side. Then begin with Exercise 12. Perform each of the walking exercises for one or two pool crossings during the first few sessions. Increase over the next weeks.

## EXERCISE 12. SHALLOW WATER WALKING—BACKWARD, FORWARD, SIDEWAYS

Walking **backward** in water is easier than walking forward, so you will start by walking backward. Face the side of the pool and prepare to take your first small steps onto the sore knee. Look to see that you have an unobstructed space behind you, then begin walking backward. Don't worry about your arms while walking backward. If you feel pain when you step on the injured knee, try the basic modifications shown in the box above. Walk slowly across the pool, turn and continue walking backwards across the pool again. Keep your steps short until you can walk without a limp, then gradually lengthen your stride. After crossing the pool several times, try walking forward.

Face the center of the pool and prepare to walk **forward**, taking a small step onto your sore knee. Hold the opposite arm forward to establish an opposition position. Take first one small step, then another, moving your arms and legs in time with each other. Once again, if you feel knee pain, try the basic modifications. Make sure your right arm moves with your left leg and your left arm moves with your right leg. If this cross-crawl patterning (see page 66) is too difficult to master right now, hold your arms comfortably to your sides for balance. Eventually you do want to learn to walk with opposition between your arms and legs, but that isn't your first priority—walking without a limp is. Cross the pool several times, walking with small steps, until any gait irregularities are gone. Then you can begin lengthening your stride.

Next walk **sideways** across the pool, starting by pushing off with your strongest side and stepping onto the sore side. Then bring the fit leg to a closed position so your feet are in line and nearly touching. Step and close, step and close, in this manner across the pool, starting with small steps. Look down at your feet. Many people incorrectly turn their feet in the direction they are stepping. However, you want to keep your feet straight forward in order to strengthen the hip abductor and adductor muscles. Constantly check your feet to make sure they are parallel and pointing straight forward. If you encounter any pain, move to deeper water, take smaller steps, or put on your flotation belt. Don't lurch or lean from side to side. Rather, keep your shoulders and hips level throughout the sideways walking. When you've crossed the pool **keep facing in the same direction** so as you recross the pool you will this time push off with the opposite leg.

### EXERCISE 13. MARCHING

Begin marching by lifting a knee to the position shown in photo 10-13A, or as high as you can before you feel increased knee pain. Lean forward and take a step, then lift the other knee up to a similar position. If you feel pain in the sore knee and you've tried the basic modifications in the box on page 173, don't lift your knee so high. Pay attention to the direction your knees are pointing while you march. Perhaps your right knee is pointing straight forward while your left knee points slightly to the left side or across the mid-line of your body. Try to correct the movement so that **both knees point straight forward**. If the correction causes increased knee pain, make note of that to tell your doctor. Continue **aiming toward** correct biomechanics but only so far as you feel a slight discomfort, no pain. Use bent arms in opposition to the bent knees. Your right arm moves in time with your left knee and your left arm moves with your right knee. When marching in this flat-footed position becomes easy, progress to marching and lifting onto your supporting foot as shown in photo 10-13B. This variation helps improve your balance and increases the strength in your calf muscles.

**10-13B**
Marching, lifting onto ball of foot with each step

**10-13A**
Marching

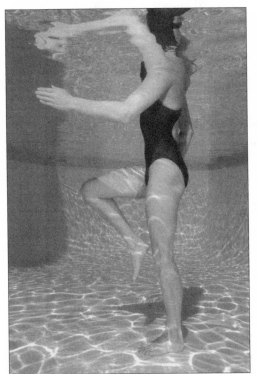

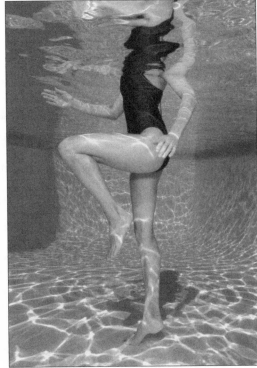

## EXERCISE 14. BOUNCING — BACKWARD, FORWARD

**Wear a flotation belt the first time you try this. When you feel confident your knee can tolerate this force, remove the belt.**

Bouncing backward is easier than bouncing forward, so start backward. Face the side of the pool, slowly bend both knees, and lower yourself to a half-squat position. Gently straighten both legs at the same time and take a small jump backward. Immediately bend both knees again and let the belt and the water catch most of your weight. Smoothly continue bouncing backward across the pool. Now try bouncing forward.

When you feel ready, try bouncing backward then forward on just one leg. Try the strongest leg first, then gently try the recovering one. If you feel pain, simply lift your leg and let the water catch you. You might not be ready for one-legged bounces yet. Try again in another week or two.

## Stretching

Stretching reduces muscle tension and makes your body feel more relaxed. It increases the range of motion of your knee joint while it helps you get to know your own body better: as you stretch, you receive messages from your body. Listen to these messages carefully.

Never force a stretch if there is pain. Stretch only to the point of discomfort to find your limit. Then ease back a bit and hold a challenging stretching position while you breathe slowly and deeply to assist the stretching process.

Turn to face the side of the pool for stretching exercises 15 to 20. You may wear a flotation belt and do them in deep water, or remove the belt and do them in shallow water.

### DOES ONE SIDE HAVE MORE RANGE OF MOTION?

Don't be surprised to find that one leg or one side of your body is more flexible or moves more easily than the other. You can address that imbalance by spending more time stretching the tighter side. The easiest way to do that is to stretch the tight side first, then the other side, then return to the tight side for a final stretch.

## EXERCISE 15. CURL AND STRETCH

With both hands hold the side of the pool, a gutter, or a ladder. Walk your feet up the side of the pool as high as you comfortably can. Bend your knees and curl in as tightly as you can without causing increased knee pain (see photo 10-15A). Tuck your chin to your chest and push your tailbone down toward your heels. Inhale and exhale slowly five times as you relax your neck, shoulders, back, and legs. Now slowly straighten your legs as far as you can, even though you may not reach the position shown in photo 10-15B. Allow yourself to experience slight discomfort, but don't push into pain. If this is too difficult, or if it causes too much pain, lower your feet until you can do the stretch. Take five slow, deep breaths. Repeat.

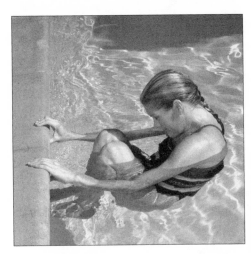

**10-15A**

Curl and stretch (Hydro-Tone belt shown)

**10-15B**

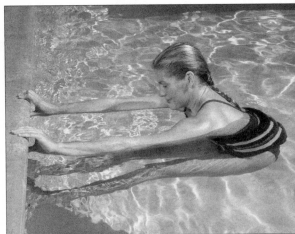

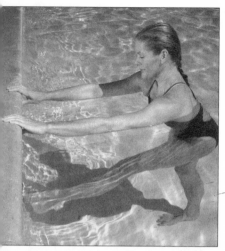

## EXERCISE 16. HAMSTRING STRETCH

Continue holding the side of the pool, a gutter, or a ladder with both hands. Place your left foot, toes up, against the pool wall as shown in photo 10-16. Keep your neck, shoulders, arms, and back relaxed throughout the exercise. Gently straighten your left knee as far as you can while you breathe deeply and slowly five times. If this is too difficult or causes too much pain, place your foot lower on the pool wall or onto a low step in the pool. Repeat with the other leg. Over the next weeks and months try to raise your foot higher on the wall and then try to push your heel to make contact with the pool wall.

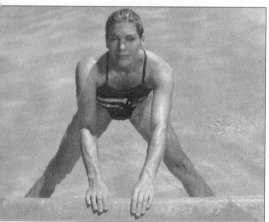

## EXERCISE 17. BODY SWING

Continue grasping the side of the pool and open your feet to slightly more than shoulder-width apart, with your feet slightly turned out (see photo 10-17A). Put your weight on the balls of your feet. Your heels don't touch the wall. Without moving your hands, bend your right knee as far as you can and swing your body to the right. Your left knee stays fully straight (see photo 10-17B). Now swing back to the left by straightening your right knee and bending your left. Slowly swing back and forth four to six times, working especially on gaining more flexion in your problematic knee at every swing. If you feel the need to stop and push into the stretch on your sore knee, do it slowly while breathing deeply.

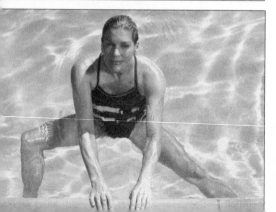

10-16 (top) Hamstring stretch

10-17A Body swing (middle photo)
(Hydro-Tone belt shown)

10-17B Body swing (bottom)

## EXERCISE 18. QUAD STRETCH

Hold the side of the pool for balance with one hand. Grasp the ankle of your strongest leg and slowly pull the heel toward the buttocks, as shown in photo 10-18. If you can't reach your ankle, try putting a strap or towel around your foot, then pull it up as far as you can without pain. Keep the knees close together and make sure you haven't gone into a "sway back" position. Breathe deeply five times as you feel the muscles relax and lengthen. Switch sides and slowly attempt this exercise on the affected knee. You may not be able to do this one right away. Ask a friend to assist you in gently bending your knee until you can finally grasp it yourself. Or use a strap or towel to work into this stretch by yourself.

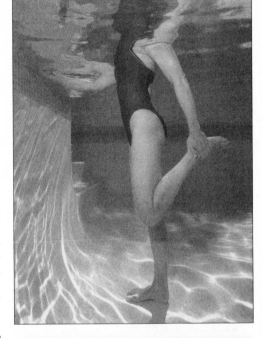

## EXERCISE 19. HIP FLEXOR STRETCH

**If you have a lower back problem, ask your doctor or therapist if you can do this exercise.**

Start in the position shown in photo 10-18. (You may be using a towel or a friend may be helping you do this stretch.) **Keep your elbow straight** as you allow your knee to swing straight backward to the position shown in photo 10-19. Look up at the ceiling to further increase the stretch of the hip flexors. Breathe slowly and deeply five times, then repeat on the other side.

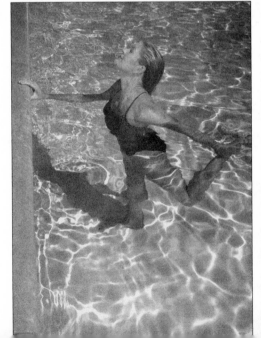

**10-18 (top)** Quad stretch

**10-19** Hip flexor stretch

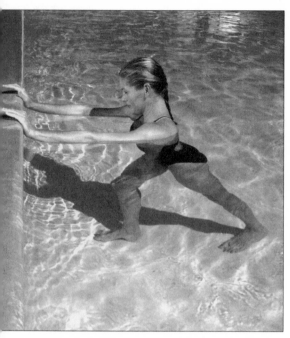

10-20 Gastroc stretch

### EXERCISE 20. GASTROC STRETCH

If you're wearing a flotation belt, remove it now and move to the shallowest part of the pool. The water's buoyancy lifts your body weight up, so you'll need to use your hands to grasp the side of the pool to push your weight downward (see photo 10-20). Place the affected leg forward with the knee slightly bent. Reach the other leg behind you, toes pointing forward, knee fully straightened. Push the heel of the rear leg toward the pool bottom and hold it there while you breathe slowly and deeply five times. Now switch legs and gently try the affected side. If this feels good, push downward into the stretch even harder. If it hurts your knee, push less or bend your knee slightly.

## Waterpower Workout Exercises

As you gain strength and flexibility in your knee, you might be tempted to return to your normal sports activities. Before you do, try these gentle impact exercises to see if your knee is ready. If you experience knee pain during or after these exercises, you aren't yet ready to return to your sport, in which your knee will face an even greater weight-bearing load. Continue to prepare your knee for land activities by increasing the number of repetitions you do of each exercise and by increasing the intensity of your running. (See Lynda Huey's *Waterpower Workout* video or *The Complete Waterpower Workout Book* for a complete series of shallow-water exercises. All products mentioned in the text are listed in the Appendix that starts on page 296.)

Wear a flotation belt the first time you try these jumping exercises. By doing so, you allow your knee to learn to exert force as you push off, but you let the belt and the water catch your body weight (instead of your knee) as you land. Start with only ten reps the first time. Then, if your knee remains painfree, add two reps each session until you've reached thirty reps. Then remove the flotation belt and start over again at ten. You'll be surprised how much more weightbearing your knee must do when you're not wearing the float belt. Work back up to thirty reps of each exercise, and then take your first try at your favorite sport or land workout.

## EXERCISE 21. LUNGES

Assume the lunge position shown in photo 10-21, with your right knee forward and bent. Your left leg is straight and to the rear. Your left arm is bent at the elbow and forward for counterbalance. Jump up and switch arm and leg positions so that the left leg is now forward and the right arm is forward. Make sure your right arm is forward with your left leg and your left arm is forward with your right leg. Each right-left cycle is one repetition.

**10-21** Lunges

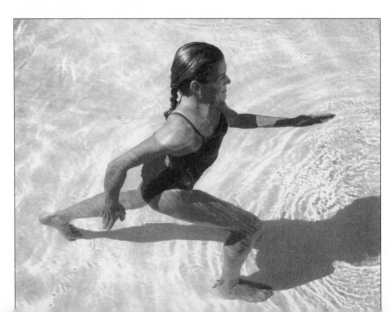

**10-22A**
Squat jumps

## EXERCISE 22. SQUAT JUMPS

Begin bouncing with your feet shoulder-width apart. Jump high and pull your legs together at the top of the jump, as shown in Photo 10-22A. Land with your feet apart (see photo 10-22B), and with your knees bent. Straighten your legs as you rise and bend them as you come down.

**10-22B**

## EXERCISE 23. BOUNCING LEG SWINGS

**If you have lower back problems, don't swing your working leg behind you as far as shown, only down to the pool bottom slightly behind you.**

Bounce on your stronger leg and hold the affected leg straight out in front of you, as shown in photo 10-23A. Reach the opposite arm forward for counterbalance. You'll stay on this one leg without touching the other leg down through the first half of your repetitions. As you bounce, swing your affected leg backward to the position shown in photo 10-23B

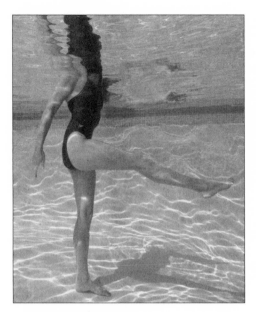

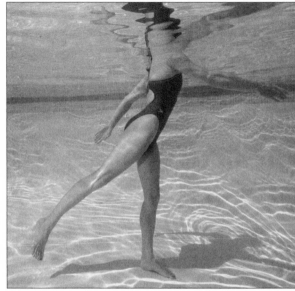

**10-23A** Bouncing leg swings          **10-23B**

on one bounce, then back to the starting position on the next bounce. Take time to make sure your arms and leg are moving in opposition and do your best to keep the knee of the swinging leg straight throughout the exercise. Next, switch legs and try this while bouncing on your affected leg, swinging the other leg forward and backward with each bounce. Finish the other half of your reps on this side if you can. If this causes increased knee pain, stop. You can try it again next week when your knee may be more able to tolerate it.

## EXERCISE 24. FRONT KICKS

Stand on your left leg with your right leg and left arm straight in front of you, which is the same starting position as shown in photo 10-23A. Jump and switch arm and leg positions so that the left leg and right arm are now held straight in front of you. Each right-left cycle is one repetition.

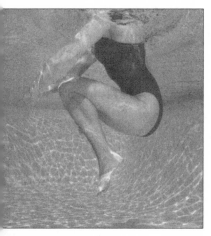

## EXERCISE 25. POWER FROG JUMPS

Bounce gently with your feet together and your arms out to your sides, at chest level. Jump off both feet and lift both knees toward your chest as you sweep both arms forward to meet in front of you (see photo 10-25). Push the arms back to their starting position as your feet return to the pool bottom.

**10-25** Power frog jumps

## EXERCISE 26. ONE-LEGGED FROG JUMPS

Bounce on your stronger leg and bend your affected knee in front of you, as shown in photo 10-26A. Hold your arms out to your sides for balance. Now push off with your weightbearing leg and lift that knee up to meet your suspended knee as shown in photo 10-26B. Then drop your working leg so the foot touches the pool bottom. Immediately bend the knee and prepare for another push-off. Do half your repetitions on this leg, then try to duplicate that same pushing and lifting movement with your affected leg. Start by sitting low in the water and barely lifting the affected knee. If your knee feels fine, start pushing off harder and standing taller in the water.

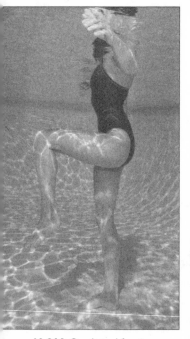

**10-26A** One-legged frog jumps

**10-26B**

## EXERCISE 27. SHALLOW-WATER RUNNING

Begin running in place, simulating good running form on land. (Do not run across the pool, because that creates entirely different forces on your body and knee.) The head and chest are erect and the eyes look straight ahead. The shoulders stay down and stable without rocking from side to side. Lift your knees and pull your arms directly forward and back without any lateral movement. Make sure you are using opposition: your right arm is forward with your left knee and your left arm is forward with your right knee.

Once you've established good running form, begin increasing your speed. If your form breaks down, slow down and correct your biomechanics. Then pick up the pace again. A work period is followed by a slower recovery period, then another work period until you've completed two to ten minutes of running. Monitor your heart-rate where noted.

Do the low-intensity intervals the first session. If they seem too easy, don't move up to moderate intensity until the next session. You won't know until tomorrow if your muscles or knee are going to be sore or if you will become overly fatigued. If you begin the medium-intensity program on your second day in the pool, and they again seem too easy, follow the same rule as before: don't move up to the high-intensity program until the next session. Wait to see how your body responds after exercise. If the low- or medium-intensity program suits you well, stick with it several weeks each before attempting to move up. It's better to make slower, steadier progress than to hurt your knee trying to do work you're not ready for. Such a mistake will force you backward for a week or even two to recover. It may have taken months or even years to develop this knee condition, and it may take you just as long to help correct it.

### Low Intensity

Run (easy), one to three minutes

Walk across the pool and back

Run (easy), one to three minutes

(Heart-rate check)

### Medium Intensity

Run (easy), one minute

Run (medium or fast), thirty seconds

Run (easy), thirty seconds

Run (medium or fast), forty-five seconds

Run (easy), thirty seconds

Run (medium), one minute

(Heart-rate check)

Repeat this sequence if you wish.

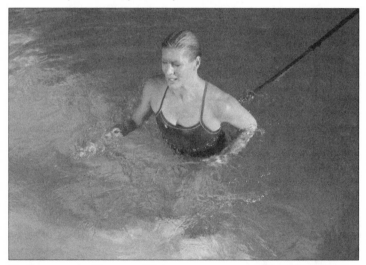

**10-27** Shallow-water running with tether

**Tether yourself to a railing or a gutter on the side of the pool when running at high speeds, as shown in photo 10-27. This keeps you stable and allows you to focus on your workload instead of constantly adjusting your position.** (See pages 151 and 152 for more about the Waterpower Workout tether.) If you can't find anything to tether to, you can tie a rope to a nearby tree or ask a training partner to hold the end.

## HIGH INTENSITY

Run (moderate), one minute
> Run (slow) thirty seconds

Run (moderate), one minute
> (Heart-rate check)

Run (fast), thirty seconds
> Run (slow), thirty seconds
> Run (fast), thirty seconds

(Heart-rate check)
Repeat this sequence.


Run (moderate), one minute
Run (sprint), one minute
(Heart-rate check)
Repeat this sequence.

---

### HELPING TO CORRECT A TRACKING PROBLEM

An elite athlete who experienced a tracking problem of her knee discovered that her knee pain went away if she stayed out of deep water. She sensed she needed impact to drive strength into her quads and she needed to avoid deep-water running, which created a "clicking" sensation at her patello-femoral joint. Here's her program:

| | |
|---|---|
| **Gait Training Warm-Up:** Exercises 12 to 14 | 2 minutes each |
| **Waterpower Workout:** Exercises 21 to 26 (First set comfortably, second set jumping higher) | 2 x 20 reps **(no belt)** |
| **Running**, Exercise 27, high-intensity program | 20 minutes |
| **Kick Training:** Exercises 8 to 11 | 1 minute each, last 30 seconds harder |
| **Stretching**: Exercises 15 to 20 | 30 seconds each |

Gradually increase the difficulty of your shallow-water interval session over the next weeks and months. If your knee doesn't object, you may decide to do **only** shallow-water intervals. Choose deep or shallow or a combination of the two as you prefer. Use what you've learned about interval training from the previous examples to create your own personalized interval session that lasts fifteen to twenty-five minutes. Vary it from day to day to avoid losing interest.

## Lower Extremity Exercises

Earlier you stretched all the major muscles that surround the knee. Now you'll be performing exercises to strengthen those same muscles. If you feel any pain during these exercises, **slow down or narrow the range of motion.** You'll start your program using only the water's resistance against your legs. As your strength improves, you can add equipment: ankle weights or Hydro-Tone resistance boots to increase the workload or a buoyancy cuff to increase your range of motion. The boots offer three-dimensional resistance: they create extra workload in every direction you move—forward, backward, sideways, up, and down. Ankle weights, while easier to put on, return you to gravity—they pull straight downward so that only your upward movements will feel increased resistance. Buoyancy cuffs lift your foot higher in the water, causing increased knee extension when doing Exercise 30 and increased knee flexion during Exercise 31.

Keep in mind that your knee may feel different every day, so you must adjust your workload accordingly. **If your knee is painful, don't use any equipment.** Save it for days when your knee and the muscles around it are feeling painfree and eager for more work.

**Start with ten repetitions of each exercise. Add two reps each session until you've worked your way up to thirty. (Or**

**follow the guidelines in Chapter 8.) Then begin adding equipment for extra workload.**

Do all the reps on your strongest side before repeating on the affected side. In this way, your involved knee can learn from the fit knee: try to duplicate the correct movement of the stronger knee. Notice if your sore knee isn't capable of as much motion as your stronger knee. In that case, you may decide to do more repetitions on the weaker side to try to bring it slowly back to full function. The easiest way to do more work on one side is to do all your exercises on the sore leg, do a second set on the stronger side, then go back to the sore side for another set.

## EXERCISE 28. LATERAL LEG RAISES

Stand with your hand on the side of the pool, facing the end of the pool (see photo 10-28A). Maintain erect posture and lift your leg directly to the side (see photo 10-28B). Don't lean to the side in order to lift your leg higher. Keep the feet parallel so that your knee and foot point forward rather than upward. Pull your leg back to the starting position.

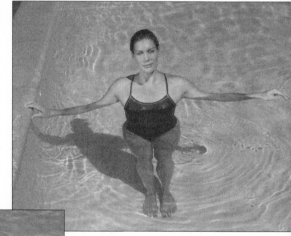

**10-28A** Lateral leg raises

**10-28B**

## EXERCISE 29. STANDING LEG SWINGS

**To protect your lower back, tighten your abdominal and gluteal muscles as you do this exercise.**

Continue standing erect with your hand on the side of the pool for stability. Swing your leg straight forward (see photo 10-29A), then swing it down and to the rear (see photo 10-29B). **If a full swing backward hurts your back, don't reach so far.**

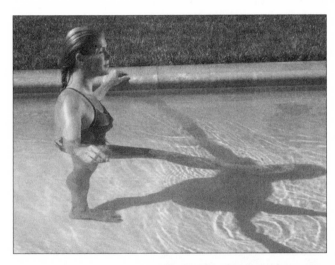

**10-29A**
Standing leg swings

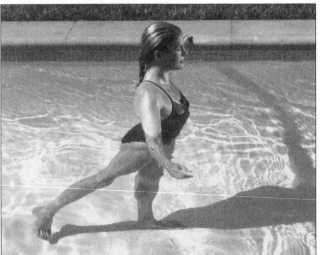

**10-29B**

## EXERCISE 30. QUAD EXTENSIONS

**Start this exercise without the equipment shown. After you've built up to thirty reps, you can add the Hydro-Tone boot.**

Hold your unaffected knee straight in front of you, with the foot aimed toward the pool bottom as shown in photo 10-30A. Kick the lower leg away (see photo 10-30B), then pull it back to the starting position. Repeat your reps on the affected knee. If this exercise causes knee pain, move more slowly, lower your knee, or limit your range of motion—straighten and bend only as far as you can without pain. Don't add the boot, an ankle weight, or a buoyancy cuff until you've progressed in strength and have been painfree at least one week.

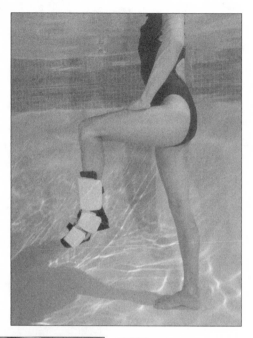

**10-30A**
Quad extensions
(Hydro-Tone boot shown)

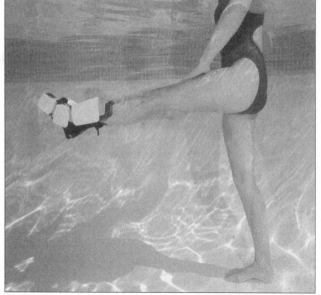

**10-30B**

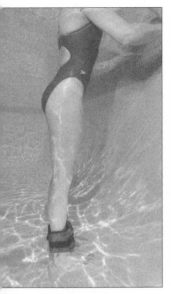

**10-31A (above)**
Hamstring Curls
(Hydro-Fit flotation cuff
shown)

**10-31B (right)**

## EXERCISE 31. HAMSTRING CURLS

**Start this exercise without the equipment shown. After you've built up to thirty reps, you can add the Hydro-Fit buoyancy cuff.**

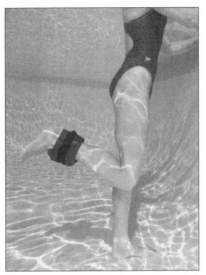

Start with your knees together, and feet together on the bottom of the pool (see photo 10-31A at left). Keep your knees together as you lift your heel toward your buttocks (see photo 10-31B) then push your foot back to the starting position. Stay within a painfree range of motion for each knee. Over time you'll be able to reach for full flexion (bending) and full extension (straightening), but maybe not the first time you try this exercise. Don't add the cuff, a boot, or an ankle weight until you've progressed in strength and have been painfree at least one week.

**10-32A**
Squats

## EXERCISE 32. SQUATS

Face the side of the pool in chest-deep water with your feet parallel and shoulder-width apart (see photo 10-32A.) Both hands grasp the side of the pool. Focus your eyes on a point directly in front of you and maintain that focal point throughout the exercise. Keep your back straight and slowly bend both knees until you've lowered your chin to the water (see photo 10-32B). Your heels will probably lift off the bottom at this point. Push your heels down as you stand up to the starting position. Once you've worked your way from ten to thirty reps, try single-leg squats (see photo 10-32C). Start with your stronger leg and do ten reps, then try another ten on your recovering knee. Continue to do thirty double-leg squats every session as you add two more single-leg squats to your program each time.

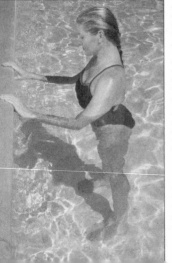

**10-32B
(left)**
Squats

**10-32C
(right)**

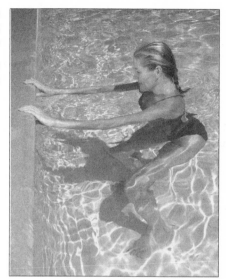

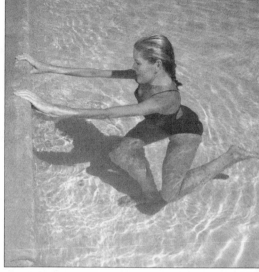

## EXERCISE 33. HEEL/TOE RAISES

Stand erect in chest-deep water facing the side of the pool. Place both hands on the side of the pool for balance. Slowly lift your heels to stand on your toes (see photo 10-33A), then slowly lower your heels to the pool bottom. Next, without changing the position of your hips, lift your toes (see photo 10-33B). Don't rock your hips backward. Make the muscles at the front of your calves do the work by maintaining proper posture.

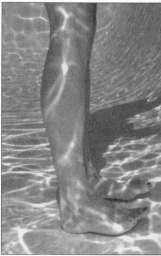

**10-33A**

Heel/toe raises

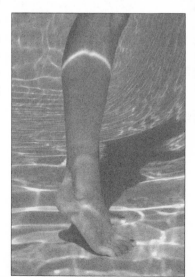

**10-33B**

## EXERCISE 34. STEP WORK

Place a pool step onto a level portion of the pool bottom at a depth where you can stand on it and still be in chest-deep water. The exercises in this series are presented in an increasing order of difficulty. Instead of starting with the unaffected knee, you'll be asked always to work your recovering knee.

**Step Up/Down.** Face the step and maintain an erect posture as you step up with your affected leg (see photo 10-34A). Then step up with your other leg (see photo 10-34B). Next, step down to the position shown in 10-34A. For example, if your right knee is the painful one, step in this manner: up right, up left, down left, down right. By stepping in this order, you do more work with your weakest knee. Do twenty up/down steps. If this is easy for you, wait until next week before increasing to thirty up/down steps.

**Stepover.** Start by stepping onto the step with your affected leg as shown in photo 10-34A. This is the only foot that will touch the step. The other foot passes over the top of the step, without stopping, and steps on the farthest side of the step, as shown in photo 10-34C. Keep your back and hips upright as you now step up and over again, returning to the starting position. If the return stepover causes increased knee pain, turn after each stepover to continue stepping forward, not doing the backward stepover yet. Start with ten reps and add two a session until you can do thirty reps. Then try the stepover-and-back again. Start with ten reps and gradually increase to thirty. When that becomes easy, step up and **stop** on the step to balance on one foot for ten seconds before continuing each stepover. Stop on top of the step both stepping over and stepping back to the starting position.

**Squats on Step.** Stand squarely on the step, with your feet shoulder width apart. Bend both knees and lower yourself to the position shown in photo 10-34D. Your heels will probably lift up. Then push back up to the starting position. Do ten reps the first day, then add two reps each session until you reach thirty.

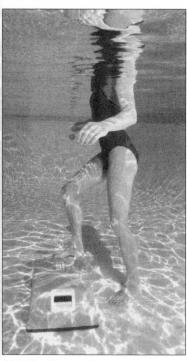

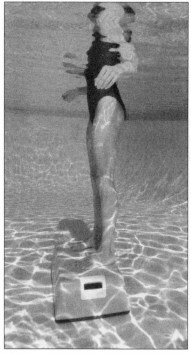

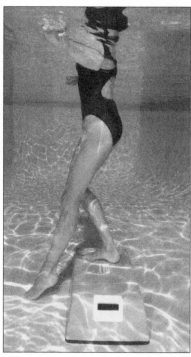

**10-34A Step work**　　　　　**10-34B**　　　　　**10-34C**　　　　　**10-34D**

The program you have just completed may be the only program you'll ever need if you're able to regain enough strength, mobility, and function to prevent the knee surgery you and your doctor thought was inevitable. Every patient would like to think he or she is a likely candidate to prevent knee surgery, but you may already have architectural damage so severe that the only solution is a restructuring of the anatomy by way of surgery. If you've accepted the fact that surgery is in your near future, you can also use this program as pre-rehabilitation to get you in shape prior to surgery. The stronger and more flexible you are when you enter the operating room, the better your body will be able to cope with the rigors of surgery and the quicker you'll return to your sports

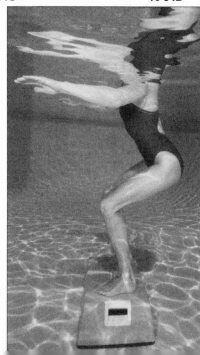

and daily activities. Further, by learning all these exercises prior to surgery, you'll find an easy re-entry to the pool at a crucial time when, if you weren't already familiar with the routine, you might shy away from it.

**If you have surgery, don't try to resume this program where you left off the week before your operation. Instead, turn to Chapter 14 for guidance on pacing your recovery correctly.**

You may be determined not to have surgery, and this program can be your key. As you work through your program, you may not know which purpose it will serve for you—prevention or prehab— and you don't need to know. Simply begin. As two to three months of diligent pool work go by, as your knee improves and your body becomes fitter, you'll find out. Don't try to figure out which path you're on after only a few weeks. You might give up too soon and jump onto the road to a surgery that could have been prevented (or at least delayed for years) if only you'd been persistent a while longer.

# 11 A LAND EXERCISE PROGRAM FOR KNEE PATIENTS

*With Tanya Moran-Dougherty, MPT*

**This chapter offers an exercise program for those who are trying to prevent knee surgery. If you've already had surgery, turn to Chapter 14 for guidelines that will lead you carefully through this program so you can protect your postsurgical knee. The ideal, of course, is to do the combined pool and land program; but if you don't have access to a pool, you can do a land-only rehab program.**

In water your knees feel better and your exercises may seem easy. So why do you need a land program at all? That is the most frequently asked question by patients who have been using the pool program to rehabilitate their knees. They say things like, "It feels like velvet when I move in the water instead of the crunch and pain of exercising on land." Or, "My knee feels so good, I wish I could stay in the pool all day." But the simple truth is that you live on land and must be able to function there. As wonderful as the water's buoyancy feels, you must eventually get out of the pool and move your knee against the pull of gravity. You need to have the strength, coordination, and balance necessary to perform your **activities of daily living (ADLs)** outside of the water. This means you need to exercise on land, where you can build the foundation of your basic functional skills, such as walking, balancing, and stair climbing.

You may have additional reasons for learning a land exercise program. You may be afraid of the water, have chlorine-sensitive skin, or not have easy access to a pool. Your goal may be to return to the gym, to competitive sports, or to recreational activities, and you want to prepare your knee for the higher impact to come. In each of these cases, you'll need a complete land-based program to rehabilitate your knee.

Different laws of physics apply on land. Instead of buoyancy and water resistance in the pool, you face the powerful downward pull of gravity on land. For instance, you don't walk the same in the water as you do on land. When you try walking in chest-deep water, you'll probably wobble at first, having to learn new balance points as you push against the water's resistance. Yet water's buoyancy takes the weight off your sore knee and allows you to stand tall and walk without limping. As you correct your gait in the gravity-reduced environment of water, you strengthen the muscles that are specific to good walking.

With that improved strength you can make the transition to land. The full transition will take time—weeks or even months, depending on the severity of your gait abnormality. When you first try to duplicate your efficient pool alignment on land, you may not be able to maintain your upright posture because your muscles aren't yet strong enough. But each time that you reinforce your proper posture in the pool, then try again on land, you get closer to regaining a normal walking pattern. **Going back and forth from pool to land allows you to take advantage of the benefits of both environments.** The water carries most of your weight while you focus on good posture and alignment; at the same time, the water's resistance forces strength into the muscles specifically used for walking. Then on land you use the strength, posture, and alignment you developed in the pool to work against gravity.

The same holds true for your other activities of daily living. As you climb stairs and perform balancing exercises in water, you have to control only a small percentage of your normal body weight because of buoyancy's upward lift. When you first try those same stepping and balancing maneuvers on land, you'll apply the skill and good form you learned in the pool, but you may not yet have enough strength to do them well. By gaining skill and strength in the pool, then transferring it to land, you'll eventually find you can perform those basic skills without a second thought to your knee. In that way, your body becomes skilled and strong in the functions necessary for your daily life on land.

Your job is to restore your ability to do the things your personal environment requires of you. For instance, if you live in a house with twelve steps, you need to be able to negotiate those steps without difficulty. You should be able to get safely into bed, the shower, and the bathtub, and in and out of the car and the easy chair. If you need to be able to perform a specific movement that wasn't offered to you in Chapter 10, create your own pool exercise to develop the skill and strength that will allow you eventually to perform that movement on land. For example, if it's difficult for you to vacuum your rug, simulate the vacuuming movement in the pool. After many repetitions, you'll be able to push and pull a real vacuum on land.

## STARTING LAND EXERCISES

Picture an astronaut on the Moon as he jumps, skips, and runs lightly across the surface in his gravity-reduced environment. When he returns to Earth, the movements he performed with such ease become harder. You'll feel the same change as you move from your pool to land program, as if you'd landed back on Earth after being on the Moon. Your body will feel heavier, and for a while you'll have to work harder to do the basic exercises that were so easy in the pool. But keep in mind that the pool program has strengthened your muscles and allowed you to relearn proper movement techniques. That strength and technique has prepared you for these land exercises that transition you to ADLs.

While you can expect some discomfort when starting these land exercises, take care not to create more pain. What's the difference? Discomfort makes you aware that there's something wrong with your knee, but pain warns you to stop what you're doing. Give your knee's monitoring system your full attention while doing these exercises, and you'll gradually increase your ability to understand the signals.

**Start with the non-weightbearing exercises only, Exercises 1 to 11.** These are the gentlest of the exercises, and all can be performed in a painfree range of motion. Stay within that painfree range and be gentle with your knee. Over the weeks, as your knee gains strength and mobility, start adding Exercises 12 to 25 as explained in Chapter 8. When you first try each of the more advanced exercises, do only two to three repetitions as a test. If you feel increased pain or instability in your knee while doing an exercise, stop. Try that exercise again next week while you continue with the exercises you **can** do without pain or instability.

---

**RED FLAGS TO STOP THE EXERCISE**
- If the exercise causes a sharp pain in your knee
- If you feel your knee "buckle" when attempting an exercise
- If the exercise causes you increased pain that is greater than "4 out of 10" on the pain scale (0 = no pain, 10 = emergency room pain)

---

During the first few weeks of this program, you may have pain in your knee **after** the exercise session. Don't worry.

Nothing's going wrong. You're reactivating something that was lying dormant, so don't let the pain alarm you. Moving your "rusty" knee is like a bear waking from its long winter nap. It yawns and growls and shows its teeth before it gets up to resume its life. Continue with the exercises, staying painfree during the session. As you do more of the exercises, you'll start seeing the results. There will be less post-workout pain and more mobility. If you suspect you need stronger motivation to follow through with your knee recovery, visit a physical therapist for precise hands-on guidance.

---

**BENEFITS OF A LAND-BASED PROGRAM**
- Increased range of motion (ROM) from the stretching exercises
- Increased strength from the exercises against gravity and Thera-Bands
- Improved balance from the balance training exercises
- Improved functional skills from the exercises that replicate basic ADLs

---

## NON-WEIGHTBEARING EXERCISES

Exercise 1 has you bend and straighten your knee both to warm up the joint and to help restore your normal range of motion. Exercises 2 to 4 are stretches for the primary muscles around the knee. Start with your fit knee to learn what is expected, then repeat the exercise with your affected knee. In all the stretches, move to a point of discomfort, then ease off just a fraction so the stretch will still be challenging, but you can still hold it for thirty seconds. While you hold the stretches, breathe deeply and try to relax further with every exhalation. Don't push yourself. A slow stretch held for thirty seconds lets gravity do the work for you. Pay careful attention to what is needed from your fit knee during the stretch so you can apply what you learn to the affected side. Then slowly, slowly attempt the stretch on the involved knee, stopping at the point you begin to feel pain. Back off just a little and breathe deeply, monitoring the amount of discomfort you feel. This will lessen over the next weeks, so pay attention.

---

**HOW MUCH KNEE FLEXION DO I NEED?**

Textbooks say the normal amount of knee flexion is 135 degrees. However, unless you're an athlete, most of your activities don't require that much flexion. Here's the minimum knee flexion you need for normal, comfortable movement:

| | |
|---|---|
| Sitting on a chair or toilet | 90 degrees |
| Getting in and out of your car | 100 degrees |
| Walking | 60 degrees |
| Negotiating stairs | 80 to 90 degrees |

---

If your knee is fairly limited in its movements, most of these stretches will be difficult at first. Don't get discouraged! You start where you start, and you progress from there. Patience and consistency are what count. Before beginning, review the guidelines in Chapter 8.

## EXERCISE 1. HEEL SLIDES

Sit erect with a towel or strap wrapped around the ball of your foot. Grasp both ends, as shown in photo 11-1A. Slowly bend your knee and use the towel to help slide your heel toward your buttocks (see photo 11-1B). Bend your knee as much as pos-

11-1A
Heel slides

sible without increasing your pain, then return to the starting position. Do ten repetitions on this side, then repeat on the other side. When this becomes easy, increase to two, and then three sets of ten repetitions.

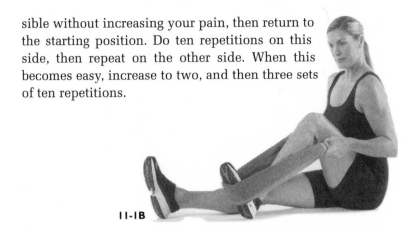

11-1B

## EXERCISE 2. HAMSTRING STRETCH

**If you have a back condition, keep one knee bent with your foot on the floor while you raise the other leg.** Lie on your back with your towel or strap still around the ball of your foot. Slowly lift your unaffected leg toward the ceiling and straighten your knee until you feel a stretch along the back of your thigh and knee (see photo 11-2). Keep your knee as straight as possible. Hold the stretch for thirty seconds while breathing slowly. When you feel the muscles relax, first try to straighten your knee more fully, then gently lift your leg higher. Repeat on your affected leg. Alternate legs until you've performed three reps of thirty seconds on each side.

11-2
Hamstring stretch

## EXERCISE 3. QUADRICEPS STRETCH

This stretch may be difficult for you to perform if you have hip pain, low back pain, or limited ROM in your knee. Three variations are listed, starting with an easy version and progressing to an advanced position. Choose the version that feels most comfortable to you while giving you the most effective stretch. If you choose version B or C but you're not yet doing weightbearing exercises, do those stretches **only** on your affected side while you stand on your stronger leg. In all three versions, do not let your lower back twist or arch.

- POSITION A. Lie on your affected side with your hips directly on top of each other. Bend your unaffected knee, bringing your heel toward your buttocks. Reach back with your top hand and grasp your foot, gently pulling your heel closer to your buttocks until you feel a stretch in the quadriceps muscles in the front of your thigh (see photo 11-3A.) Breathe slowly and deeply as you hold the stretch for thirty seconds. When you feel the muscles relax, gently increase the stretch by bending your knee more. Do this stretch three times on each leg.

**11-3A**
Quadriceps stretch

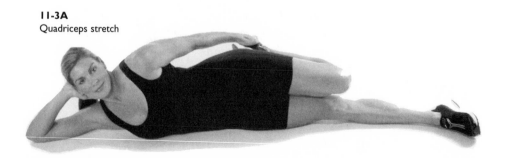

- POSITION B. **Do this exercise only on your affected knee until you progress to weightbearing exercises.** Stand approximately one foot in front of a chair, with your back facing the chair. Place the foot of your affected leg on top of the chair (see photo 11-3B). You should feel a stretch along the front of your thigh. If you don't feel a stretch in this position, move one to two steps away from the chair. Hold the stretch for thirty seconds. Do this stretch three times on your affected side only until you progress to the weightbearing exercises. Then, alternate legs until you've done three stretches on each leg.

11-3B

- POSITION C. **Do this exercise only on your affected knee until you progress to weightbearing exercises. If you can't reach your ankle, you're not ready for this exercise. Start with versions A or B instead.** Stand behind a chair with one hand touching it for balance. Reach back and grasp the ankle on your affected side, as shown in photo 11-3C. Pull your heel toward your buttocks until you feel a stretch in your quadriceps. Breathe slowly and deeply as you hold the stretch for thirty seconds. When you feel the muscles relax, gently increase the stretch by bending your knee more. Do this stretch three times on your affected side only until you progress to the weightbearing exercises. Then, alternate legs until you've done three stretches on each leg.

11-3C

## EXERCISE 4. GASTROC STRETCH

Start with Position A while you're doing only non-weightbearing exercises. Once you add weightbearing exercises to your program, try version B. Then choose the version that feels most comfortable to you while giving you the most effective stretch.

- POSITION A. Sit tall with both legs straight in front of you. Start with your unaffected leg. Place a large bath towel or belt around the ball of your foot and grasp both ends. Keep your knee straight, then pull the ends of the towel toward your abdomen until you see your toes point toward your torso and feel a stretch along the back of your knee and calf (see

**11-4A** Gastroc stretch

photo 11-4A). Hold the stretch for thirty seconds. Alternate legs until you've done three reps on each side.

11-4B

- POSITION B. **Don't do this exercise until you're ready for weightbearing.** Stand facing a wall, with your feet shoulder-width apart. Place both hands on the wall at shoulder level. Keep your toes pointing forward as you move the foot of the affected leg forward and the other foot back. Lean your body into the wall, keeping your back leg straight and your heel on the ground (see photo 11-4B). You should feel a stretch in the calf muscles of your straight leg. If you don't feel a stretch, move your feet further away from the wall. Hold the stretch for thirty seconds. Repeat by moving your affected leg to the rear stretching position. Alternate legs until you've done three reps on each side.

Exercises 5 and 6 are isometric exercises that help you build strength in your quadriceps and hamstrings without requiring any movement of your knee joint. Exercises 7 to 11 are active motion exercises that keep you non-weight-bearing while you focus on restoring active strength in the muscles that surround your knee and the hip. (See muscle groups on pages 35 and 47.)

If you have osteoarthritis, a meniscus tear, or a tracking problem, you may be skeptical that a strengthening program can help. You would be correct if you assumed that exercise can't cure osteoarthritis. However, certain prescribed exercises can help correct a tracking problem, prevent further deterioration of cartilage, restore ROM, and strengthen the knee enough to support a healing meniscus tear. (Remember the analogy of the gardener turning a painful blister into a pain-deadened callus? See page 92.) Further, strong muscles will absorb forces acting on the knee joint and help to support the ligaments around the joint.

**Do all your sets and reps with your stronger knee first, then repeat with your most affected knee.** Try to duplicate with your affected knee the good movement patterns of your stronger knee. Your goal is to reach equal strength and flexibility in both knees. Thus, if you strengthen and stretch one knee, you must also strengthen and stretch the other. Give your fit knee a moderate amount of workload to keep it functioning and strong while you work the unfit knee to its maximum so it can begin to "catch up."

**Start with one set of ten reps. When one set is no longer challenging, increase to two sets of ten reps. When two sets become easy, increase again to three sets. Alternate legs so one leg can rest while the other leg is working.**

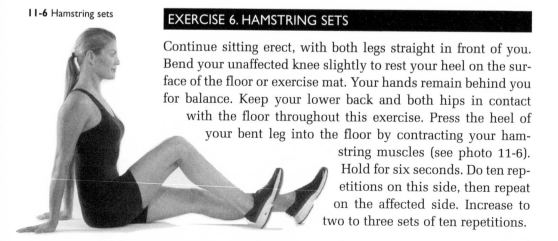

## EXERCISE 5. QUAD SETS

Sit erect, with both legs straight in front of you and your hands behind you for balance. Roll a small hand towel and place it under your unaffected knee (see photo 11-5). Keep your toes pulled back toward your head. Tighten your quadriceps muscles while pushing the back of your knee into the towel. You should see your kneecap move slightly toward your hip if performing this exercise correctly. Hold for a count of six and slowly release. Do ten reps on this side, then repeat with the affected knee.

**11-5**
Quad sets

- **If you have patellofemoral problems,** you may feel pain doing this exercise. In that case, roll a larger towel to place under your involved knee. If your pain continues with each muscle contraction, try this: Gently tighten your quads and press down until you reach the point where you feel pain, then back up slightly into your painfree range and hold for a count of six. You may not be able to do ten reps the first week, but do as many as you can without increasing your pain. Try to add at least two reps each exercise session.

**11-6** Hamstring sets

## EXERCISE 6. HAMSTRING SETS

Continue sitting erect, with both legs straight in front of you. Bend your unaffected knee slightly to rest your heel on the surface of the floor or exercise mat. Your hands remain behind you for balance. Keep your lower back and both hips in contact with the floor throughout this exercise. Press the heel of your bent leg into the floor by contracting your hamstring muscles (see photo 11-6). Hold for six seconds. Do ten repetitions on this side, then repeat on the affected side. Increase to two to three sets of ten repetitions.

## EXERCISE 7. STRAIGHT LEG RAISES

Lie on your back, with your affected knee bent and your unaffected knee straight. Pull your toes toward you and tighten the quadriceps on your unaffected leg (see photo 11-7A). Place your hands palms down next to your legs for support. Keep your lower back and both hips in contact with the floor throughout this exercise. Keeping your knee straight and your quads tight, slowly lift your leg to the level of your bent knee (see photo 11-7B). Slowly lower your leg to the starting position. If you perform this exercise correctly, you should feel your calf touch the floor before your heel. Do ten repetitions on this side, then repeat on the affected side. Increase to two to three sets of ten repetitions.

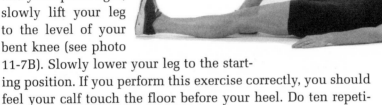

**11-7A**
Straight
leg raises

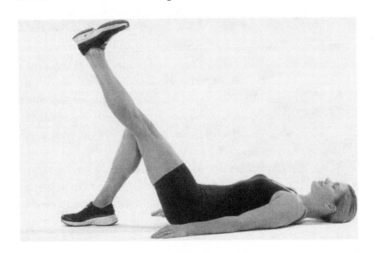

**11-7B**

## EXERCISE 8. HIP ABDUCTION

Lie on your affected side, with your hips directly on top of each other and legs straight (see photo 11-8A). Keep your knees straight and toes pointed forward throughout this exercise. Slowly lift your unaffected leg toward the ceiling without rotating your leg outward (see photo 11-8B). Return to the starting position. Do ten repetitions on this side, then repeat on the affected side. Increase to two to three sets of ten repetitions.

**11-8A** Hip abduction

**11-8B**

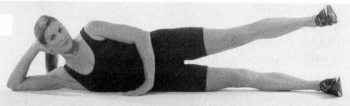

## EXERCISE 9. HIP ADDUCTION

Lie on your unaffected side, with your hips directly on top of each other. Bend your affected knee and place it on the floor in front of you as shown in photo 11-9A. Keep your unaffected knee straight and toes pointed forward. Slowly lift your unaffected leg toward the ceiling without rotating your leg (see photo 11-9B). Return to the starting position. Do ten repetitions on this side, then repeat on the affected side. Increase to two to three sets of ten repetitions.

**11-9A** Hip adduction

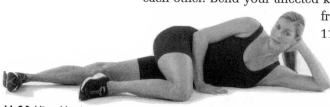

**11-9B**

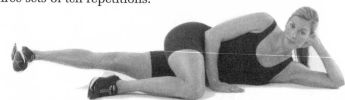

## EXERCISE 10. HIP EXTENSION

**Skip this exercise if you have a low back condition**. Lie on your stomach, with your arms folded and your chin resting on them as shown in photo 11-10A. Lift your stronger leg slowly toward the ceiling while keeping your knee completely straight (see photo 11-10B). Avoid twisting your hips or arching your back. Do ten repetitions on this side, then repeat on the affected side. Increase to two to three sets of ten repetitions.

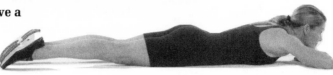

**11-10A**
Hip extension

**11-10B**

## EXERCISE 11. QUADRICEPS EXTENSION

Sit in a chair, with your feet flat on the floor and your hands beside you for balance (see photo 11-11A). Slowly straighten your unaffected knee by tightening the quads (see photo 11-11B). Return to the starting position. Do ten repetitions on this side, then repeat on the affected side. Increase to two to three set of ten repetitions. If your sore knee hurts too much during this exercise, don't fully straighten it, but move through a pain-free range.

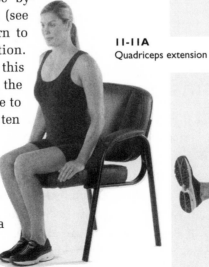

**11-11A**
Quadriceps extension

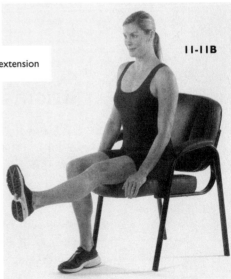

**11-11B**

**11-11C**
Quadriceps
extension
for VMO

- **If you have patellofemoral problems,** modify this exercise to **focus on the VMO** (see page 50). Sit in a chair as described in Exercise 11. Place a ball or pillow between your knees (see photo 11-11C). Squeeze the ball or pillow while slowly straightening your unaffected knee (see photo 11-11D). Focus on the quad muscles on the inner portion of your knee. Increase to two to three sets of ten repetitions. Do ten repetitions, then repeat with the affected knee. If your sore knee hurts too much during this exercise, don't fully straighten it, but move through a painfree range.

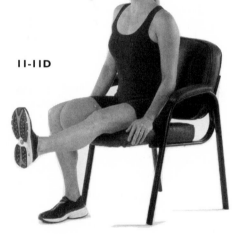

**11-11D**

## WEIGHTBEARING EXERCISES

In order to function fully in your normal daily routine, you need to be able to carry your body's weight easily throughout the day. Exercises 12 to 15 are designed to strengthen the muscles that surround your knee as you lift, balance, rise, lower, and bend. **If you feel increased knee pain or feel as though your knee is going to "buckle" while doing an exercise, skip it. Wait another week before trying any difficult exercise again, but continue doing the ones you can.**

## EXERCISE 12. HAMSTRING CURLS

Stand, holding the back of a chair or a table for balance. Bend your unaffected knee by bringing your heel toward your buttocks (see photo 11-12). Don't let your working knee drift forward. It should stay in line with your standing knee. Focus on your hamstring muscles as they lift your heel. Do ten repetitions on this side, then repeat on the affected side. Increase to two to three sets of ten repetitions.

**11-12**
Hamstring curls

## EXERCISE 13. TOE RAISES

**11-13**
Toe raises

Stand flat on both feet as you continue holding the back of a chair or a table for balance. Slowly rise onto the balls of your feet as shown in photo 11-13. Do not lean on your arms or use them to pull yourself up. Repeat this exercise for ten repetitions. Increase to two to three set of ten repetitions.

## EXERCISE 14. SINGLE LEG STANCE

**11-14**
Single leg stance

Continue holding the back of a chair or table for balance. Shift your weight onto your stronger leg and bend your affected leg (see photo 11-14). Balance on one leg as long as possible (up to thirty seconds) with only a light touch on the chair for balance. Repeat this exercise on the affected leg. Go back and forth until you've done five repetitions on each side. Once this gets easy, keep your hands several inches away from the chair and touch it only if you begin to lose your balance. If you have good balance, try this exercise with your eyes closed, but keep your fingertips resting on the chair or table for safety.

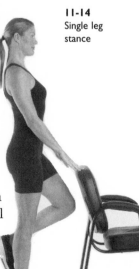

## EXERCISE 15. SINGLE TOE RAISES

This is an advanced version of Exercise 13. Once you've mastered the single-leg stance of Exercise 14, try single toe raises, performing the exercise on just one foot at a time. Start in the position shown in photo 11-14, then rise to the position shown in Photo 11-15.

# FUNCTIONAL TRAINING EXERCISES

By doing the weightbearing exercises, you became able to support your body weight on one leg. That skill alone is invaluable, for it allows you to walk with a correct gait pattern and perform other functional activities, such as putting on your pants while standing. Now, by adding functional training Exercises 16 to 21, you'll refine your skills so you can better control your body's weight as you lower yourself into and rise from a chair, as you bend forward to perform daily chores, and as you go up and down stairs in a reciprocal pattern.

## EXERCISE 16. WALL SLIDES

Lean your back against a smooth wall, with your feet shoulder-width apart and approximately two feet in front of you. Use your arms to brace yourself so you feel secure. Your toes point forward throughout this exercise. If you're positioned properly, as shown in photo 11-16A, your knees will never move in front of the line of your toes. Keep your back flat to the wall and slowly lower your body down the wall, toward a sitting position. Stop if you feel increased knee pain. (You may not be able to lower yourself as far as the 90-degree position shown in photo 11-16B. Stop wherever your knees tell you to.) Return to the starting position and repeat until you've performed ten reps. Increase to two to three sets of ten repetitions. After you've mastered three sets of ten reps, work toward reaching a full sitting position of 90 degrees.

11-16A
(left)
Wall slides

11-16B
(right)

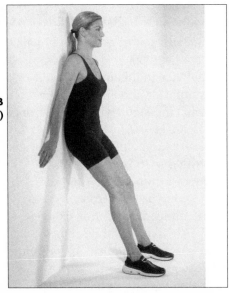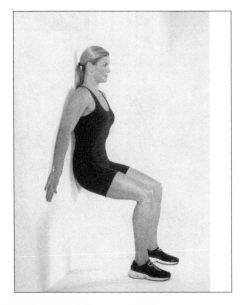

## EXERCISE 17. GOOD MORNINGS

11-17A
Good mornings

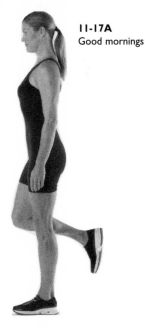

Stand on your unaffected leg and slightly bend your affected knee, as shown at right in photo 11-17A. Focus your eyes on a point on the wall in front of you. Keep your back straight, with your hands to your sides as you slowly lean forward to the position shown in photo 11-17B. If you can go all the way to a 90-degree bend, do so. Return to the starting position. If you have difficulty balancing, lightly place your fingertips on the back of a chair while you gain both balance and strength. Try again without holding onto anything next week. Repeat ten times on this leg, then do ten reps on your affected leg. Increase to two to three set of ten repetitions.

11-17B

11-18A
Step-ups

## EXERCISE 18. STEP-UPS

Stand in front of a four-inch stair, step stool, or a large book. **If you have problems with balance, hold onto a counter or dresser for support.** Maintaining an erect posture, step onto the stool with your stronger leg (see photo 11-18A). Don't let your hips sway to the side to help you step up. Next bring the sore leg onto the step (Photo 11-18B). Step down, leading with your sore leg first. This stepping pattern protects your affected knee as you learn to do this exercise. Do ten repetitions like this, then repeat with the opposite stepping pattern: up with the sore, up with the strong, down with the strong, down with the sore. This pattern makes you work your affected knee more. Increase to two to three sets of ten repetitions. When three sets of ten reps becomes easy, use a six to eight-inch step or a higher stack of books.

11-18B

## EXERCISE 19. SIDE STEP-UPS

Stand next to a four-inch stair, step stool or large book. Step sideways onto the stool with your stronger leg (see photo 11-19A). Bring your sore leg onto the step (see photo 11-19B). Step off the stool with your sore leg, then bring your stronger leg down to the floor. Do ten repetitions like this, then repeat with the opposite stepping pattern: up with the sore, up with the strong, down with the strong, down with the sore. (You'll start on the opposite side of the step.) This pattern makes you work your affected knee more. Increase to two to three sets of ten repetitions. When three sets of ten reps becomes easy, use a six- to eight-inch step or a higher stack of books.

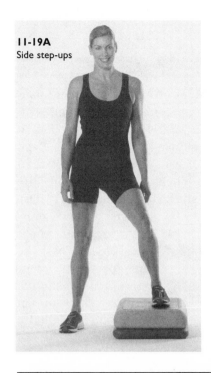

**11-19A**
Side step-ups

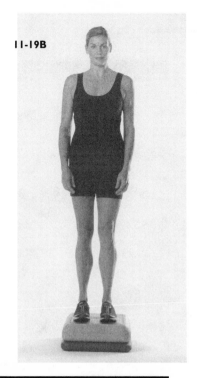

**11-19B**

## EXERCISE 20. SINGLE LEG WALL SLIDES

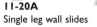

This is an advanced version of Exercise 16. Start in the same position as shown in photo 11-16A. Now lift your affected leg off the floor several inches by bending your knee (see photo 11-20A). Slowly lower yourself toward a sitting position, keeping all your weight on the stronger leg (see photo 11-20B). Return to the starting position. If this exercise is too difficult, modify it by lowering toward a sitting position with **one leg** then pushing yourself back to the starting position with **both legs.** Do ten repetitions on this side then repeat on the other side. Increase to two to three sets of ten repetitions.

**11-20B**

**11-20A**
Single leg wall slides

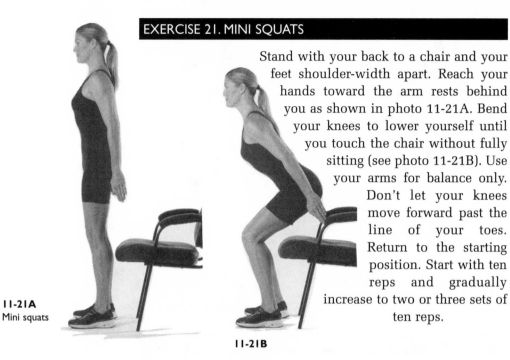

**EXERCISE 21. MINI SQUATS**

Stand with your back to a chair and your feet shoulder-width apart. Reach your hands toward the arm rests behind you as shown in photo 11-21A. Bend your knees to lower yourself until you touch the chair without fully sitting (see photo 11-21B). Use your arms for balance only. Don't let your knees move forward past the line of your toes. Return to the starting position. Start with ten reps and gradually increase to two or three sets of ten reps.

11-21A
Mini squats

11-21B

## THERA-BAND RESISTANCE EXERCISES

Stretchy latex bands can be used to create resistance and increase your workload. Thera-Bands are six inches wide and come in standard colors that designate their graded resistance. Yellow is the easiest to stretch, then red, green, blue, and gray, in increasing order of resistance. Extra resistance makes your muscles work harder, and they quickly gain strength. In Exercises 22 to 24, you'll tie the band into a loop. Exercise 25 requires an untied Thera-Band.

As you gain strength each week, you'll progress through the Thera-Bands as shown in the box on page 219. Move from the yellow to the red Thera-Band only when the exercises become easy and you need more resistance. Use that same criteria to move to green, then blue, then gray.

## STEPS IN THERA-BAND PROGRESSION

| | |
|---|---|
| Yellow: | 1 set of 10 reps |
| | 2 sets of 10 reps |
| | 3 sets of 10 reps |
| Red: | 2 sets of 10 reps |
| | 3 sets of 10 reps |
| Green: | 2 sets of 10 reps |
| | 3 sets of 10 reps |
| Blue: | 2 sets of 10 reps |
| | 3 sets of 10 reps |
| Gray: | 2 sets of 10 reps |
| | 3 sets of 10 reps |

## EXERCISE 22. TERMINAL KNEE EXTENSION WITH THERA-BAND

Stand behind a chair, with your hands holding the back of the chair. Place the tubing around one of the chair's legs and behind your unaffected knee as shown in photo 11-22A. (You can place a small hand towel behind your knee for comfort.) Position the resistance tubing so that it is parallel with the floor. Take a step back until you feel tension on the Thera-Band. Begin with a slight bend in your unaffected knee. Then tighten your quads and straighten your knee against the Thera-Band (see photo 11-22B). Don't move your hips to help straighten your leg. Do ten repetitions on this side, then repeat on the affected side. Increase your resistance and sets as suggested by the table above.

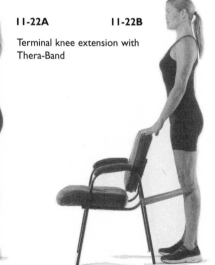

**11-22A**     **11-22B**

Terminal knee extension with Thera-Band

## EXERCISE 23. QUAD EXTENSIONS WITH THERA-BAND

**11-23A**
Quad extensions
with Thera-Band

Sit erect in a chair and wrap a loop of Thera-band around both your ankles, as shown in photo 11-23A. Fully straighten your unaffected leg to the position shown in photo 11-23B. Do ten repetitions on this side, then repeat on the affected side. Increase your resistance and sets as per the table on page 219.

**11-23B**

## EXERCISE 24. HAMSTRING CURLS WITH THERA-BAND

**11-24A**
Hamstring curls
with Thera-Band

**Do this exercise *only* on the affected side.** Continue sitting upright with a loop of Thera-Band around both ankles. Straighten your legs as shown in photo 11-24A. Bend your affected knee, pulling your heel toward your buttocks (see photo 11-24B). Return to the starting position. Do ten repetitions. Increase your resistance and sets as per the table on page 219.

**11-24B**

## EXERCISE 25. MINI-SQUATS WITH THERA-BAND

Stand on an untied length of Thera-band, with your feet shoulder-width apart. Bend your knees to a partial squat position and grasp the Thera-Band so you can feel the tension in the band as shown in photo 11-25A. Rise against the resistance of the Thera-band to the position shown in photo 11-25B. When you squat, don't let your knees move forward beyond the plane of your toes. Do ten repetitions. Increase your resistance and sets as suggested by the table on page 219.

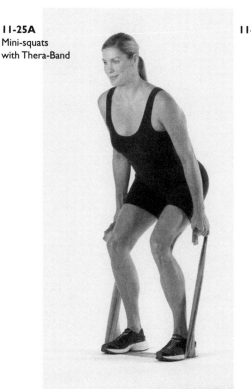

**11-25A**
Mini-squats
with Thera-Band

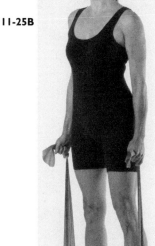

**11-25B**

# 12 KNEE SURGERY

This is the chapter we hoped you'd never have to read!

If you've put forth serious effort in a pool program, a land program, or in both, but believe you haven't made significant improvement in your knee's condition, you may need to confront the idea of surgery. You're probably taking pain medication, but your discomfort continues to wake you in the night. You may have reached the point at which, because of pain, you can no longer face your daily physical activities. You may even have consulted a surgeon and been told that you should plan to have knee surgery.

**TRY TO POSTPONE SURGERY**

The improvement of technology is a good reason to try to postpone surgery. We **all** hope for a more elegant and holistic solution to knee problems, and every day brings us closer. It's possible that in five or ten years we might not be doing knee surgeries this way. There may be a laser procedure that's appropriate or an ultrasonic tool that can destroy spurs the way we crush kidney stones. We may develop the perfect cartilage-enhancing substance to inject directly into the knee joint, a product that, despite the ad campaigns of drug companies, is **not** here yet. Even further into the future, gene therapy may eliminate many knee conditions before they happen.

Although the surgical case studies we discuss in this chapter took place in the operating room at Cedars-Sinai Hospital in Los Angeles, you can be assured that surgeries similar to these take place in hospitals in New York, Seattle, Chicago, Atlanta, and elsewhere in the United States.

We offer this chapter in hopes that reading the experience of another patient with a similar diagnosis to yours will make the thought of your operation less frightening. Four case studies follow, one for each of these surgeries:

- Meniscus
- Tibial plateau fracture
- ACL reconstruction
- Implant (total knee, unicompartmental, etc.)

## MENISCUS SURGERY

A thirty-year-old computer engineer was playing tennis when he planted his foot for a forehand stroke and felt a sharp pain in his knee. He stopped playing, returned home, and iced his knee twice that day. His knee didn't swell and the pain subsided slightly over the next few days. Then, while driving home less than a week later, he noticed he couldn't straighten his knee fully. Later that evening he found himself limping because of a knife-like, stabbing pain on the inner portion of his knee joint.

Meniscus tears can be small or large, and they can occur in many different shapes and angles. While most meniscus tears happen immediately and rarely progress to anything more serious, a bucket-handle tear can develop when the initial rip is large in area and further activity displaces the cartilage. In this case, the torn part of the patient's meniscus flopped open into the joint and this "bucket handle" acted like a doorstop blocking the full motion of his knee joint. (See illus. 3-3 on page 42.)

Meniscus surgery is performed through an arthroscope. *Arthros* in Latin means "joint," and *scope* means "to look inside." During knee arthroscopy, I make a tiny puncture wound and insert a pencil-sized optical device into the knee joint. A miniature television camera attached to the arthroscope allows me to view the interior of the joint on a large monitor.

Before arthroscopic procedures became available in the 1970s, open procedures were necessary to work inside the knee joint. Those open procedures meant cutting through the skin and the underlying tissues, which was costly in terms of tissue damage. Further, it was common practice in those days to remove the entire meniscus, something we now know accelerates the degeneration of the knee. Today's tiny instruments inserted into the knee joint allow us easily to reach inside the knee to view the meniscus damage, then determine whether to try to repair the torn portion or, if that's impossible, to trim it out.

Photo 12-1 was taken through an arthroscope looking inside his knee joint at the time of surgery. Compare it with photo 12-2, a normal medial meniscus. Since this patient's meniscus tear included the white-white zone (see page 31),

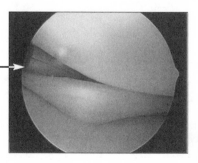

**12-1**
The arrow points to a long bucket handle tear in a meniscus as seen through the arthroscope.

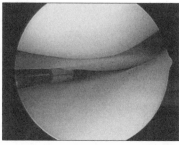

**12-2**
A surgical tool lifting a normal meniscus as seen through the arthroscope.

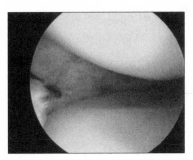

**12-3**
The patient's meniscus after the torn portion was trimmed out, leaving the rim of the memiscus intact.

there was virtually no chance the meniscus would heal if we tried to repair it. Photo 12-3 shows his meniscus after the torn portion was trimmed out, leaving the rim of the meniscus intact. If the tear had been in the red-red zone (see page 31), we could have placed sutures in the meniscus and over the next six weeks the meniscus would have healed.

This patient can now move his knee fully. He returned to his sports as soon as he was comfortable doing so. Because no cortisone was injected into his knee, his recovery was "real" and not masked by medicine. Be sure to tell your surgeon you don't want cortisone injected into your knee during surgery or post-operatively.

## TIBIAL PLATEAU FRACTURE

A forty-year-old man was skiing through some trees when he hit a bump and fell. He felt a pop in his knee, felt severe pain, and was unable to stand on that leg. His leg was put in a splint by the ski patrol so no further damage or displacement could occur. Then he was taken to the local emergency room, where X rays confirmed a fracture of his tibial plateau. His knee was treated with ice. A CT scan was also ordered, as is appropriate for a fracture to the tibial plateau. The CT scan shows if the crack or fracture is severe enough to require surgery or whether it can be treated by placing the patient in a brace and on crutches with no weightbearing for six weeks.

In this case, the fracture was displaced enough to warrant surgery. If it hadn't been repaired, this patient certainly would have been left with an uneven surface to his knee's cartilage that would prematurely wear out and lead to swelling, pain, and poor alignment—the cardinal signs of posttraumatic osteoarthritis (see page 53).

Until recently, when faced with a tibial plateau fracture, we had to open the skin and muscle with a three to six-inch incision to expose the bone, then use tools to squeeze the bone back together. We did a bone graft, stuffing the new bone into the space beneath the flat surface and holding the whole thing together with plates and screws. (See the X ray in figure 12-4A.) Now, through a half-inch incision and under X ray guidance, we can fire two pins horizontally across the tibia just below the tibial plateau. Those pins serve as guide wires over which we next place two screws, like threading two pencils over their own lead that had been removed. Through an arthroscope in the joint, we can watch as the screws advance, pushing and squeezing the two pieces of the tibia together to mesh correctly. We no longer violate all the tissue that used to be damaged when inserting a plate and six screws. In that older method of repairing a tibial plateau fracture, the hardware might later need to be surgically removed if the patient complained of soft-tissue pain where perhaps the tip of a piece of metal was sticking

**12-4A**
In the old style of repairing a tibial plateau fracture, major damage was done to the surrounding tissues in order to insert a plate and six or more screws.

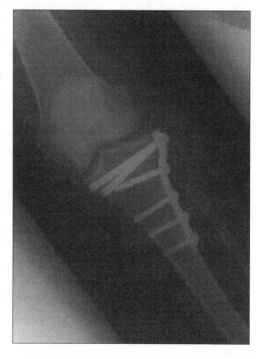

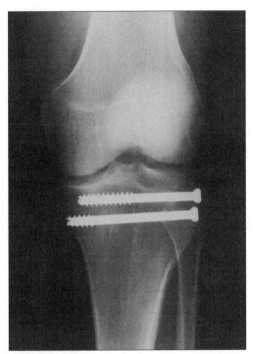

**12-4B**
The current style of repairing a tibial plateau fracture shoots two pins across the tibia then threads two screws over them causing minimal tissue damage.

into a muscle, causing inflammation. The new, minimally-invasive technique makes recovery and healing easier for the patient. The X ray in figure 12-4B shows the current, less-invasive technique.

This patient left the hospital in two days and has returned to all his activities, including skiing. His hardware is painless and therefore no second surgery will be needed to remove the two screws.

## ACL RECONSTRUCTION

A thirty-five-year-old actress who enjoys playing basketball on the weekends jumped for a rebound. When she landed on her defender, she heard and felt a pop in her knee, which immediately became swollen. She limped off the court and immediately iced and elevated her knee. An MRI confirmed the diagnosis of a torn anterior cruciate ligament (ACL).

The tremendous beauty of the knee's engineering is at stake whenever an ACL is reconstructed. I've learned that as a surgeon I'd better put the new ligament exactly onto the footprint of the original ligament—I have to place both ends of the new ACL exactly where it originated and inserted—in order for the patient to have a knee that has full motion and full stability. Patients who have difficulty bending and straightening their knees after ACL surgery are often fighting the fact that their surgeon didn't put their ligament exactly where it was supposed to be. I've found that by using the magnified field of the arthroscope to view inside the knee, I can locate exactly the former location of the knee's torn ligament.

This patient and I had to choose a new ligament to graft inside her knee. Since Gore-Tex and other synthetic grafts have gone out of favor, there are currently three choices: 1) cadaver, which is called an allograft; 2) her own hamstring tendon; or 3) her own patellar tendon. Using her own hamstring or patellar tendons is called an autograft. The allograft uses tissue from a donor while the autograft moves the patient's own tissue from one site to another. The harvesting of a hamstring tendon is less invasive and requires less healing time than the harvesting of the patient's patellar tendon.

---

### MY CHOICE OF GRAFT FOR ACL

Even though cadaver tendons are tested carefully for HIV and hepatitis, there have been cases where people have contracted those diseases from their allographs in ACL surgery. When the hamstring tendon is used as a single strand, it is weaker than an ACL, so surgeons will double, triple, or even quadruple the strands to increase its strength. Given those facts, I prefer the patellar tendon for what, in my opinion, is the safest, strongest ACL reconstruction. If your surgeon suggests cadaver or hamstring grafts, make him give you a legitimate reason for his choice. Ask the right questions: "What about the contamination issue in cadavers?" "What about the strength issue with the hamstring tendon?" You'll have a fundamentally different operation, depending on your surgeon's choice, and you have the right to know why he or she has made that choice.

---

The ACL ligament contains a large blood vessel which, when torn, spills blood into the joint; hence, the immediate swelling. In the days before the MRI (see page 122), we would aspirate the joint by sticking a large needle inside

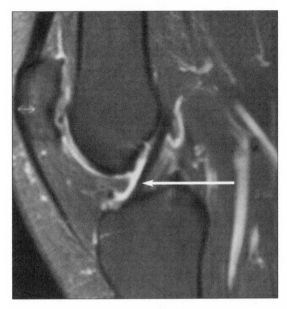

and withdrawing fluid to see if it was bloody. If blood was present in the joint fluid, we diagnosed a torn ACL. Nowadays, the MRI is an accurate and less painful way of looking inside the knee to make the diagnosis of a torn ACL.

Figure 12-5 is an MRI of a normal, intact ACL. Photo 12-6 shows the patient's torn ligament. Notice the frayed strands and bruised structures. Photo 12-7 shows the new ligament in place after ACL reconstruction surgery. A portion of the patient's patellar tendon was used to replace the ACL.

**12-5**
The arrow points to an intact ACL in an MRI of a normal knee.

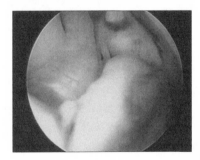

**12-6**
The patient's torn ACL. Note the frayed strands and bruised structures.

**12-7**
The new ligament in place after ACL reconstruction surgery.

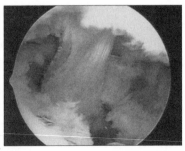

This patient has returned to all sports without restrictions. I made a custom brace for her when she was three months post-op. She used the brace for one full year during sports in which she pivoted, such as tennis, skiing, and basketball. The brace did not give stability so much as the psychological security of reminding her to think twice before moving her knee. Further, wearing the brace warned those around her to respect her space.

## KNEE IMPLANT SURGERY

A fifty-five-year-old business executive retired to play golf and tennis. As he increased his weekly hours of recreational activity, he noticed that his knee was painful and swollen. Eventually his play was curtailed by his knee's loss of motion from the swelling. Going up and down stairs had become difficult, and the Advil and Aleve he was taking no longer brought him pain relief. He went through a three-month pool program in an attempt to prevent surgery, and he felt much stronger from doing the exercises. But he still had more and more pain, even at rest. His X rays appeared in Chapter 6, showing the classic signs of osteoarthritis (figures 6-2A and 6-2B on pages 120 and 121):

1. Joint space narrowing
2. Spurs (osteophytes)
3. Cysts (black holes in the bone)
4. Sclerosis (whiter bone where the pressure on the bone is increased)

This patient opted to have knee implant surgery. The X rays in figures 12-8A and 12-8B on page 232 show his knee after surgery. Notice that the medial and lateral ligaments, patella, and muscles are all preserved. We spare as much bone as possible in this modern surgical technique.

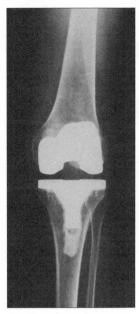

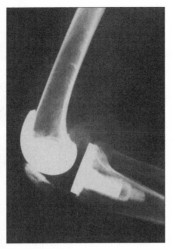

The ACL and PCL are removed and the cartilage is replaced. You can see the metal and plastic coating the ends of the bone where the cartilage used to be.

He was out of the hospital in three days and returned to the pool for six weeks of post-surgical therapy. Six months after surgery, the patient returned to golf and tennis. He is once again enjoying the leisure he worked so hard for in his retirement.

**12-8A** (above)
The front view of a knee after total knee surgery

**12-8B** (above, right)
The side view of a knee after total knee surgery

## RESPECTING AN OLD INCISION

If you had previous knee surgery, perhaps an open meniscectomy or a fracture surgery, expect your surgeon to use the previous incision site when opening your knee. By extending your old incision slightly into new territory, your doctor can acquaint himself with what your normal tissue anatomy should be. In scar tissue everything looks the same: thick, white, and compacted, with no distinguishing features. If your surgeon doesn't extend your incision slightly past the compacted scar tissue, he won't be able to look into the healthy tissue to learn where the nerve is running and where the planes and layers of normal tissue are situated—it would be like flying a plane into a cloud without radar. You don't want to run into something you can't see. You want your doctor to see all the vital tissues surrounding your previous scar to determine where the nerves and blood vessels enter that amorphous clump of scar tissue so he won't inadvertently damage them.

# 13 IN AND OUT OF THE HOSPITAL

If you've never had an operation, or never spent time in a hospital, you'll have dozens of questions, concerns, and, yes, fears as you prepare for knee surgery. In this chapter we'll try to allay such fears and quiet your concerns by giving you enough information to feel like a veteran on your arrival at the hospital.

One of the first things you can do is talk directly to another of your surgeon's patients who has successfully gone through the whole process. I make that easy in my office by having a list of patients who are good at articulating what happened to them. I've got a range of ages and personality types on the list, so if I have a patient who is a very active woman in her fifties who wants to return to tennis, I look at my list and match her up with someone who had similar thoughts and goals. I match women with women and men with men, and I do my best to match their diagnoses exactly. If you have arthritis, a torn ligament, a torn meniscus, one knee, two knees, an additional back or hip problem, you should speak to someone else who has gone through the same surgery. My new patient may have questions she isn't comfortable discussing with me, such as "When can I get up by myself to go to the bathroom again?" or "When can I have sex again?" It's also important for patients to ask such questions as, "Am I going to be able to get in touch with the doctor after surgery?" "Is his or her bedside manner genuine?" What was your relationship like with the doctor in terms of care before, during, and after the surgery?" Talking these things over with an "experienced" patient can give you valuable information and reassurance.

If you'll be having a meniscectomy or other arthroscopic procedure, you'll check into the hospital and be released on the same day, thus becoming classifed as a true outpatient, someone who doesn't spend the night. In recent years, the definition of an outpatient has been stretched to meet the criteria and payment fees established by most insurance policies, which define an outpatient as someone who stays in the hospital under twenty-four hours. Thus, if you're having an ACL reconstruction, you may be classified as a twenty-three-hour outpatient and spend the night in the hospital. Only if you're having total knee surgery will you become an inpatient and stay several days in the hospital.

## PRIOR TO SURGERY

Between the time your surgery is scheduled and the date of the surgery itself, there are several things you can do to help ensure the best possible outcome.

VISIT AN INTERNIST OR YOUR FAMILY DOCTOR. Although internists, family practice doctors, and general practitioner doctors are slightly different, all look at your overall medical condition. About a week before your scheduled operation, you'll have a general physical exam to make sure that you're a safe candidate for surgery. The doctor will test your heart and lungs and take blood tests and a chest X ray. All of these pre-op tests make sure you're fit for the surgery and the anaesthesia.

If you don't have your own medical doctor, or if your doctor doesn't practice at your surgeon's hospital, your surgeon should certainly recommend one for you.

**PREPARE YOUR HOME FOR YOUR RETURN.** Especially if you live alone, you must have things prepared in advance. You'll be on crutches, a walker, or a cane at first, so think about what belongings would be hard for you to reach in your daily life and move them to a more convenient position. If your chairs are low, pile one cushion onto another to make it easier for you to sit and rise from your chairs. Consider having meals already prepared and in your freezer, and groceries in your cupboards. Move comfortable clothes to the front of your closets. Look at your bathroom and consider adding safety bars near the toilet and in the shower or bathtub.

**PRE-OP EDUCATION CLASS FOR KNEE IMPLANT SURGERY INPATIENTS.** If you'll be an outpatient for a meniscectomy or an ACL reconstruction, you'll have such a short hospital stay that you won't need the pre-op class to teach you about your daily hospital routine. Instead, you'll generally receive a phone call from a surgical nurse twenty-four to forty-eight hours prior to your surgery to verify your medical history and your allergies, to remind you not to eat or drink anything as of midnight the night prior to surgery, and to ask you to bring to the hospital a list of the medicines you're currently taking and the amount you take daily.

Many hospitals have a pre-op education class for their total knee surgery patients. If yours doesn't, you'll get a mini version of such a class right here in this chapter, a comprehensive preview of what's to come. If your hospital **does** have a pre-op class, you'll most likely meet a surgical nurse and a physical therapist who will talk you through your entire stay in the hospital. You'll learn about anesthesia, painkillers, the use of walkers and crutches, and what to expect during each of your days in the hospital. You'll also be presented with a vital idea regarding your long-term recovery: **the success of your surgical outcome will depend on you—how hard you're willing to work at your rehabilitation will dictate the amount of movement you regain in your new knee.** Because the knee is such a complex joint with multiple ligaments, menisci, and muscles, it requires in-depth strengthening and stretching. You're going to have to work through the pain right away or it can freeze up, leaving you with a knee that barely bends and straightens. The pre-op class prepares you mentally for the work you have ahead.

**DONATE BLOOD PRIOR TO KNEE IMPLANT SURGERY.** For most knee surgeries, we work with a tourniquet on the thigh, so there will be little bleeding and little need for you to receive blood during the operation. But if your surgeon thinks it's necessary for your specific operation, you'll want to donate blood designated for your own use prior to surgery. The standard practice for a total knee surgery is two pints, but check with your doctor. Family members might want to donate blood for you, which is admirable, but even if they're the most clean-living people you know, they may have picked up something unbeknownst to them just by eating in a restaurant. The big worry with blood transfusions, of course, is HIV, but you could also be exposed to hepatitis or other infectious diseases from someone else's blood. There's no question that the safest blood to get if you lose blood during surgery is your own.

Talk to your surgeon about the issue of donating blood, then find out which blood bank works with your hospital and contact it. A transfusion specialist will see you and go over the details. Generally the blood can be stored for about six weeks before surgery. I tell my patients that once they pick a surgical date, they can count back from that date.

Give a pint of blood, wait a week, rest, give a second pint of blood, wait a week, rest, then have the surgery. In a time that can be filled with anxiety, it's good to do things in a smooth, orchestrated fashion.

UNDERSTAND YOUR INSURANCE BENEFITS. During your stay in the hospital, you'll want to devote your time and effort to healing. This means you should do all the research about your insurance well before your operation.

Many of today's health plans use various "networks," groups of health-care providers that contract with your hospital. Your surgeon and the hospital you choose may both be part of your network, but many of the services they'll use are not. The anesthesiologist is a medical doctor who administers and supervises the anesthesia, the drugs that will sedate you or make you unconscious. The anesthesiologist who usually works in the operating room with your surgeon might not be part of your network. The lab that does your urine and blood work might not be either. If you go blindly into surgery without researching, you'll receive bills from companies you've never heard of after the surgery. Many of them won't be part of your network and that will trigger a different, and probably higher, deductible on your insurance. **Take the time to find out exactly what services you'll need for the surgery and what companies you can select that are part of your network**. This can save you hundreds of dollars. You may, however, decide to keep your doctor's "team" together. For instance, if the anesthesiologist who usually works with your surgeon in the operating room isn't in your network, you may decide their close working relationship is worth the extra money.

In particular, you should know what your post-hospital benefits are. Does your insurance pay for home care or an extended care facility? Your doctor wants you well taken care of, and he might say, "Since you don't have anyone at home to help, we'll send you to this extended care location." But your insurance may not pay for the place he has in mind.

Find out what equipment your insurance will pay for. The physical therapists in the hospital will teach you how to use crutches, a cane, or a walker safely. You'll continue to need those crutches, cane, or walker when you first leave the hospital. If you're over 5'6", you'll find that a raised toilet seat will be safer and more comfortable to use than having to lower yourself onto a standard-height toilet. You'll use one in the hospital, and you'll be given one to take home as well. The hospital staff will do their best to verify what will be paid for by your insurance, but you should know, too. If they send you home with equipment that won't be paid for by your insurance, you will be paying for it.

## DAY OF SURGERY— CHECK-IN

Operating rooms generally open around 6:30 a.m., so your arrival time might be quite early. Find out about parking in advance. You don't want to be late because you couldn't find a parking place. More and more surgeons are asking all their morning patients to arrive between 6:00 and 6:30 a.m. and all their afternoon patients to arrive around 10 or 11 a.m. This practice allows surgeons to change the order of surgeries if it becomes necessary due to an emergency, the need to wait for specific sterilized surgical equipment, or the last-minute arrival of results from a medical test. If someone else's surgery is cancelled or delayed at the last minute, you could be whisked off into the operating room early. On the other hand, an operation might take longer than was expected, and you could go into surgery late. The timing of your surgery depends on what happens to the patients in your designated operating room. More than one surgeon may be sharing the room that day, so the timing doesn't always depend on your doctor alone.

Bring a book or magazine to read, since you could have a long wait. I tell my patients, "Do you want to rush to the airport just a few minutes before the plane, or do you want to get there with plenty of time and relax until the plane takes off?" You want to minimize stress on the day of your surgery any way you can, so try to be early and relax in the waiting area reading something you enjoy.

Using a felt-tip pen, write NO on your knee that isn't having surgery. This is standard practice in orthopedics, where we have two arms and two legs, unlike other surgeries where there is only one gall bladder or one heart.

Wear casual, loose-fitting clothing that won't press against your incision site on your return home. Wear a comfortable pair of shoes that you can slip into easily without bending to put them on.

Study the following checklist. Then, when you talk to that other patient who's had surgery similar to yours, ask if there was anything unique about your particular hospital. Was there anything he or she forgot to bring from home that would have made the hospital stay more pleasant?

## CHECKLIST: WHAT TO TAKE TO THE HOSPITAL

- A list of the medications you're currently taking and the amount you take daily of each. Don't bring the actual medications with you. The hospital will supply them for you.
- Pajamas, a robe, slippers, glasses, hearing aid, dentures, and personal toiletries such as your toothbrush, hairbrush, shampoo and deodorant.
- Insurance information.
- Emergency phone numbers.

- Your cane, crutches, or walker, if you use them. Label them with your name. If they're misplaced while you're in surgery, they can easily be returned to you.

- A copy of your advance directives. These are written statements such as a living will or health care power of attorney. They communicate your wishes for your health-care if you are unable to communicate those wishes for yourself. Advance directives forms are usually available through your hospital.

- Don't bring anything of value into the hospital the day of surgery. You don't want to lose something you cherish.

- Bring only a few dollars cash. Don't bring credit cards with you.

- Leave all jewelry at home.

### IF YOU CHECK INTO THE HOSPITAL ALONE

A growing number of people don't live with family members and are therefore responsible for their own health care, even during the difficult days of surgery. Many questions and logistical challenges will present themselves, so we've offered some suggestions.

- Bring a **copy** of your driver's license and insurance card with you when you check in, not the actual documents.

- Take a taxi or have a friend drop you off at the hospital, since you won't be able to drive yourself home.

- If you'll be staying a few days, try to make arrangements for a friend or neighbor to bring your favorite bathrobe, pajamas, shorts, or other necessities on the second or third day. You'll be wearing a hospital gown the first day or two.

- Leave your favorite wristwatch at home. Some rooms don't have clocks, so you may want to bring an inexpensive wristwatch.

## DAY OF SURGERY—ADMISSION

You'll start at the admissions desk, where there will be a list of all the people having surgery that day, so they'll be expecting you. A hospital employee or volunteer will take you to your next stop, which in most hospitals is a lobby-like waiting area for surgery. A nurse will take you into a nearby room to take your blood pressure and review any requests your surgeon may have made. You'll return to the waiting area until your surgery is ready to begin. If friends or family accompany you, they'll remain in the waiting area.

## DAY OF SURGERY—THE PRE-OP HOLDING ROOM

When it's time for your surgery, you'll be called back into the pre-op holding room where you'll change into your hospital gown. It will button or tie in the back. Your clothes will be placed in a bag. If someone is with you, this is when you'll give them all your belongings, including your wristwatch, rings, and other jewelry. If not, your bag will be locked in a special closet until you've arrived in your room after surgery. Later that day these belongings will be brought to you.

The surgical staff will settle you onto a gurney (a stretcher on wheels), and make final preparations for surgery. The nurses in the pre-op room will introduce themselves. They'll always tell you what they're going to do before they do it.

If you wear glasses, contact lenses, a hearing aid, or dentures, you'll keep all of these in place until the last minute. In the past, nurses took everything from you that was removable, but now the physicians and the nurses want patients to be as normal as possible—talking, hearing, and seeing until just before the surgery. Glasses and hearing aids are labeled with the patient's name and returned right after the surgery.

If your contact lenses are disposable, throw them away in pre-op. Bring your glasses, because you may not feel well enough to put contacts in your eyes the first few days.

The anesthesiologist will talk to you about the history of any previous surgeries you may have had. If you had trouble with nausea or vomiting, this is the time to speak up, because the timing of your antinausea medicine can be changed. If you take the medicine prior to surgery rather than after you have your first bout with nausea, you won't get as sick or possibly you won't get sick at all. If this is your first surgery, but you easily get car sick or sea sick, you might be a candidate for the antinausea medicine. Talk to the anesthesiologist about the possibility of this kind of prophylactic medicine; that is, medicine taken before it is needed to prevent something.

The anesthesiologist will place a needle in your arm to begin the intravenous fluids. You'll hear this referred to as an IV. The fluids are composed of a salt-water solution called saline, potassium, and sometimes vitamins. The IV's purpose is to give you the fluids your body would normally have or need. If your doctor ordered it, the anesthesiologist will give you a dose of antibiotics prophylactically. The length of time your IV remains in place will depend on your surgery. If you're an outpatient, nurses in the recovery room will check your blood pressure and other vital signs, and assuming everything is fine, your IV will be removed before you go home. If you're an inpatient, your IV will normally stay in until post-op day 2 or 3, because it has these additional important functions: 1) it delivers antinausea or pain medication, 2) it delivers extra fluids to bring down a fever,

3) it delivers nutrition if you aren't eating well, and 4) it delivers blood should you need a transfusion.

Just prior to surgery, I always visit my patients to help set their minds at ease. It's a tense moment, so I like to touch my patients, see their families, and make them smile in the pre-op area. **No anaesthesia or painkillers are given to my patients before I see them prior to surgery.** I like to know they're wide awake and can show me which knee we're operating on. I don't want to meet them in the operating room when they've already got their IV in and there's any hint that they aren't fully alert. As my own reinforcement, I hand-carry my patients' charts with me from my office to the operating room and I read them the morning of the surgery. I do everything possible before every surgery to ensure no mistakes are made.

---

**A VISIBLE SIGN OF AGREEMENT BETWEEN PATIENT AND SURGEON**

Our policy at Cedars-Sinai is to ask our patients to write a large "X" on their skin above the surgery site with a magic marker. The doctors initial near the X to verify they've double-checked the side of the body that needs surgery. (This procedure is now recommended by the American Academy of Orthopedic Surgeons.)

---

Someone from the surgical staff will pick you up from pre-op. They'll wheel you on your gurney into the operating room. If you'll be having a general anesthesia, you won't remember much of this part, because the anesthesiologist will have already started giving you medicine to calm you and start to put you to sleep. (Occasionally, people say they remember being moved from the stretcher to the operating table or they remember the lights, but usually they don't.)

Some people get a regional rather than a general anesthetic. You and your doctor will determine which anesthesia will be best for you.

## Preventing Blood Clots

There are inherent risks of undergoing even the smallest surgery, and you need to discuss them with your doctor. There's a risk you could have a negative reaction to the anesthesia. There's the risk of damage to the nerves or the blood vessels, since we're working so close to them. There's the risk of infection. But of all the possible complications that can happen from surgery, the most important is a blood clot, because it can kill you.

When we talk about a dangerous type of blood clot, we're talking about a clot developing in a vein in either of your legs. It sits there and then all of a sudden—right after surgery, the next day, a week later, a month later, or three months later — it lets loose and throws itself into the bloodstream and flows up to the lung. That blood clot lodges there and blocks off a part of the breathing area of that lung. If it's a big clot, you can try to breathe all you want, but there won't be an exchange of oxygen and you could die. A blood clot in a vein is called a deep vein thrombosis (DVT), while a clot that travels from one place to another is called an embolism. A clot that sticks in the lung is called a pulmonary embolism. No matter what they're called, we want to avoid all of them, so we take many precautions. We try to thin the blood immediately after surgery with anticoagulants: aspirin, Lovenox, Fragmin, or Coumadin. It's controversial which of these to use, but it's not controversial that you have to do something. Ask your surgeon what he or she uses.

During surgery, we use various medications to keep a patient's blood pressure low, and we try to finish the surgery quickly. After surgery, we try to get the patient upright as soon as possible. We use a pressurized stocking, which is placed on your non-surgical leg in the operating room and attached to an air-pump machine. When the machine pushes air into the stocking, it gently squeezes first your ankle, then your calf, then your thigh. Then the air is completely released for a few seconds before starting the massaging effect again—ankle, then calf, then thigh. The stocking essentially milks the blood out of the veins and keeps the circulation going so the blood doesn't collect in the veins. Further, the mechanical effect of squeezing the leg damages the inner lining of the blood vessels and sets in motion a chemical reaction, releasing the body's natural anticoagulants that help prevent blood clots from forming. Such squeezing doesn't have to take place over an entire leg. New "foot pumps" that squeeze only the foot are enough to stimulate the body's anticoagulant production. Many hospitals have begun using these foot pumps because they're less cumbersome and because they're cooler than stockings. Studies show that both inflatable stockings and foot pumps prevent a large number of clots during the first seventy-two hours after surgery. Ask your doctor what his routine is or what his hospital staff does.

After knee surgery, you'll have swelling in your ankle, your foot, and maybe your whole leg, because we've blocked the normal flow of fluids upstream. The swelling could last for days, weeks, or even months. During that time, you'll probably want to buy some support stockings to help manage the swelling.

---

**SWELLING TIME BY SURGERY TYPE**
- Meniscus surgery or other arthroscopy: approximately 2 weeks
- ACL reconstruction surgery: approximately 1 month
- Knee implant surgery: approximately 3 months

## CPM Machine

CPM stands for the Continuous Passive Motion machine. It's called "passive" motion because the machine bends and straightens your knee with no effort on your part. Following ACL or total knee surgery, you would be unlikely or unable to do movements needed to keep the muscles loose as well as force nourishment into the cartilage that is fed only by movement. Hence, the CPM machine was developed. You lie on your back with your leg cradled in foam-like cushions beneath your thigh, calf, ankle, and foot. The unit is open along the top surface and is held in place by velcro straps across the shin and thigh. A hinge at the knee allows a small motor to bend and straighten your knee to the exact number of degrees as specified by your surgeon at the speed requested. For example, your doctor might want your knee to bend from 0 degrees to 60 degrees eight times per minute. Since doctors have different strategies for using the CPM, ask your doctor about his plan so it won't be a surprise. You may be doing something different than other patients in the hospital, and you'll want to know why.

The use of this machine and when to begin its use is controversial. Proponents of the CPM say you'll regain your knee motion sooner if you use it. Hospitals that are trying to minimize costs will point to studies showing that a year after total knee or ACL surgery, the range of motion will be the same whether you use the CPM or not. However, the CPM may have benefits that go beyond the published studies, such as keeping down swelling, simply because you have to be lying flat to use the machine, and thus you have your leg elevated more hours during a day than if you weren't using it. I believe it comes down to a personal preference for both the surgeon and the patient. Some patients want to be left alone after significant surgery; others want to gain the confidence that comes with "doing something."

If your doctor uses the CPM, you'll begin its use in the hospital, usually six to eight hours a day. Then it will go home with you, and you'll use it as your doctor orders.

## Knee Brace

If you've had ACL surgery, you'll need protection for your newly attached ligament. You'll be put in a hinged brace that allows bending and straightening, but protects the knee from making inadvertent rotational movements that could pull on the fixation site of the new ligament. You'll sleep in the brace at night for protected movement and greater comfort. The brace has locking hinges so the surgeon can stipulate how much movement he wants for each postsurgical knee. (For the first week, I generally lock the brace so the patient can move the knee from full extension—0 degrees—to 90 degrees.) This bending and straightening hinge motion of the knee is relatively safe for ACL patients right away. You can even remove the brace when sitting, using a stationary bike, or while using the CPM machine, but don't rise from your couch, or chair, or bed, or bike without putting your brace on, because you could easily pivot when making those moves. **Remember: No pivoting!**

## Knee Immobilizer

If you've undergone knee implant surgery, you'll have no restrictions to your movements—no ligaments were attached that need to be protected and, further, your new implants are virtually bionic. But you'll likely have pain, so I place my total knee patients in a knee immobilizer at night to keep the leg fully straight, which reduces muscle spasms and the pain that accompanies muscle spasms. During the daylight hours, you'll walk without the immobilizer, do other physical therapy, and be placed in the CPM machine, but at night you'll probably be more comfortable resting in the knee immobilizer.

## Patient-Controlled Analgesia (PCA)

Patient-controlled analgesia is a device that's pre-programmed by your physician and attached bedside to the IV. It allows you to administer pain-killing drugs directly into your own IV. The program is set for a specific quantity of medicine that can be administered only once every pre-set time period, say every eight or ten minutes. ACL and meniscus patients generally aren't in the hospital long enough to use the PCA, but if you'll be an in-patient, ask your surgeon if he recommends your using the PCA.

## Exercises

Besides the passive exercise the CPM machine provides, you'll need to perform many active exercises to strengthen your knee, and they will begin almost immediately. Right after surgery, the nurses will ask you to do some ankle pumps. They'll say, "Push your toes away, then pull them back toward your head." They want to make sure you have control of your muscles and that all of the nerves are functioning. Ankle pumps also help blood flow in the legs. You're going to have pain while doing your exercises, so anticipate it: premedicate. For example, take your pain medicine before you begin your physical therapy exercises so you'll never have to play "catch up" with the pain, because then it's harder to control. If your pain meds are "on board" before you begin exercising, you'll work through the pain more easily. This concept of premedicating before exercise applies to both the PCA while you're in the hospital and to the oral medications you'll take at home.

## DAY OF SURGERY—IN YOUR ROOM

From the operating room, you'll be taken to the recovery room. If you had meniscus surgery, the nurses there and your anesthesiologist will decide when it's time for you to be discharged to go home. **If you've had meniscus surgery, skip to GOING HOME on page 253.**

The type of graft your surgeon chooses for an ACL reconstruction will determine your length of stay in the hospital. (See page 229 regarding the three types of ACL grafts.) **If yours was a cadaver or hamstring graft, you'll likely go home the same day as surgery. Skip to GOING HOME on page 253.** If your surgeon did a patellar tendon ACL graft, you may be sent to your specified hospital room for an overnight, twenty-three-hour stay.

If you're spending one or more nights in the hospital, your IV will still be in place. You'll probably be given a few more doses of antibiotics through it. Your reaction to anesthesia can give you a dry mouth and a feeling of being dehydrated. Some patients aren't nauseous at all from the anesthesia and are hungry right after surgery. They can actually start eating in the recovery room. Most patients, however, will start with liquids first, then advance fairly quickly. Their first meal might be dinner the same evening as the surgery.

Your bed will have a frame around it; knee implant patients will have a trapeze overhead. The trapeze is a hanging bar you can grasp with your hands so you can use your arms to help adjust the position of your body. As you progress, you'll use it getting in and out of bed.

---

**RESEARCH YOUR HOSPITAL ROOM**

Every hospital is different. Some have single rooms, others have two or more patients per room. Some have cable TV, some don't. Some allow you to place a cot for a visitor in your room, others do not. Do your research well ahead of surgery if those details concern you. You want to avoid a major surprise during the crucial days of recovery in the hospital.

---

You'll need to take some deep breaths to keep your lungs working well. The number one reason for a fever right after any kind of surgery is because of atelectasis, a collapse of the small airways in your lungs. That collapse can cause a fever that could lead to pneumonia, if not managed correctly. You need a good expansion of your lungs, and just being told to breathe deeply isn't enough for knee implant patients. An incentive spirometer is a device that was created to motivate patients to breathe deeply. Essentially it's a plastic toy. You'll use your own breath to move three balls to the top of the device and hold them there a few seconds. You get visual feedback about how deeply you can breathe and hold that deep breath. You'll do that several times an hour whenever you're awake. It's a wonderful way to keep your lungs clear following the anesthesia required for surgery. (ACL and meniscus patients aren't in the hospital long enough to use the spirometer.)

## POST-OP DAY 1— KNEE IMPLANT PATIENTS

It's important to me that I see my patients early the next morning, and I'm hoping your surgeon will do the same. When I make rounds (visits to all my patients in the hospital), I spend time with the patients going over exercises they can do in bed. I explain how important it is to have their brain start talking to their muscles right away. Don't think of this bed time as being "flat on your back," but as time you can use. You've been flexing and pointing your feet. The physical therapist will teach you how to do "quad sets," which are isometric muscular contractions of the front of the thigh without any movement of the knee or hip. The therapist will also start gently bending and straightening your knee for you. When you're alone, keep trying to move your leg, and soon you'll no longer be afraid of moving it. If you watch TV, do these movements during the commercials and the repetitions will add up. Then you won't be so wobbly when you stand up to walk, because your brain has already been communicating with your muscles. Before lunch, the therapists will help you up to try to sit for thirty to forty minutes.

Surgery is a pre-meditated trauma to the body. All the structures that have been cut—the skin, the muscles, the tendons, the ligaments, and bone—need time to heal. As we close the tissues following surgery, the muscles, tendons, and fascia are overlapped and held together with sutures. However, those sutures are as weak as thread; they aren't worth anything in terms of structural strength. By following your doctor's instructions regarding a knee brace or a knee immobilizer, and by limiting your exercise to appropriate movements until these tissues have fused, you won't be pulling on the repair sites where the sutures hold the tissues together. Even the incision site on the surface of your skin needs protection. If you make movements that tug on the skin, it may seep a clear fluid and delay the healing process. You want to keep the incision area dry for its smoothest healing.

## TWENTY-THREE-HOUR STAY OUTPATIENTS (SOME ACL PATIENTS)

The physical therapist will see you the morning after your surgery and start you on some exercises if your doctor has ordered them. The occupational therapist will begin teaching you how to accomplish the tasks of daily living without traumatizing your knee. She'll show you how to bathe or shower and how to use the long-handled devices that help you put on your shoes and socks. Any concerns you have about functioning in your home environment will be discussed, and she'll help solve those specific details. Your IV will be removed, you'll learn to use crutches, a cane, or a walker. Then you'll go home. If you were using a CPM machine in the hospital, it will also go home with you.

You'll see your doctor is his or her office a week later to have the bandage and stitches removed. **Skip to GOING HOME on page 253.**

## THE REST OF POST-OP DAY 1— KNEE IMPLANT PATIENTS

Although you may wish to do nothing but rest, the physical therapists have specific goals for you even the first day after surgery. They will help you sit up on the edge of your bed and dangle your legs over the side. Next they'll help you stand and balance on crutches or a walker. Most people will start with a walker the first day and graduate to crutches when they feel less wobbly or nauseous. You'll be putting weight on your postsurgical knee the day after surgery. If you managed sitting and standing relatively easily, you'll next be guided to take a few steps on your walker or crutches to the nearby chair. Practicing this maneuver from the bed to the chair is called transfer training. You'll sit in the chair for thirty to forty minutes, then transfer back into bed.

If you don't make it into the chair on the first try, the therapists will do everything possible to see that you make it on the second try later in the day. The success of your surgery will be that much greater the sooner you get going.

## THE REST OF YOUR HOSPITAL STAY

You could go home as early as day 3 or day 4. In order to be discharged, however, you have to have achieved certain goals. If you live alone, you must be able to perform all of the functions by yourself. If you have someone at home who can help you, you have to be able to do them with minimal assistance.

You'll be evaluated to see if you meet the criteria for discharge. Assuming you do, your dressing will be changed just before you leave the hospital. You'll leave that dressing in place until you visit your surgeon in his office, usually a week later.

---

**OUT OF THE HOSPITAL SOONER**
New products are emerging that function similar to a biological Crazy Glue. Instead of using sutures or staples to close a wound, we'll apply the new adhesives and, in an instant, achieve the bonding of the tissues that would normally take ten days to realize. This instant wound repair will protect against infection, decrease the time you're in the hospital, and help you begin moving more quickly.

---

## GOING HOME

MENISCUS SURGERY OR OTHER ARTHROSCOPY. You can expect that your IV will be removed in the recovery room and you'll go home the same day as surgery.

ACL SURGERY. If your surgeon did a cadaver graft or a hamstring tendon graft, you can expect to go home the day of surgery. If your surgeon did a patellar tendon graft, you will probably be discharged the day after surgery, but less than twenty-four hours after you were admitted to the hospital.

KNEE IMPLANT SURGERY. The therapists will make sure you can get out of bed by yourself and can walk to the bathroom and more than 100 feet alone before you can be discharged to go home. You'll also need to be able to walk up and down however many steps you'll be dealing with at home. If it's time for you to leave the hospital, but you're not doing these things, arrangements will have to be made for you to go to a rehabilitation facility, such as a skilled nursing unit where patients don't need medical attention but rather focus on doing intensive physical therapy twice a day while they have someone cooking their meals and caring for them.

Once you arrive home, a physical therapist or an occupational therapist will visit to see if he or she has any suggestions for making your home more efficient with your temporary limitations. If they see anything of concern, they'll make adjustments. Their goal is to make your home a safe environment while you recover from knee implant surgery.

---

**POSTSURGICAL EMERGENCIES**

If anything in your recovery is not going in a routine fashion, that qualifies as an emergency. Call your surgeon's office manager, speak to the doctor, and go in immediately. Not tomorrow, today! Even if your doctor is in the operating room, he or she can see you between cases, usually within a few hours.

These are clear-cut orthopedic emergencies:

- The wound is draining.
- The bandages have come undone.
- You've gotten your brace wet.
- You've taken a fall from your crutches.

> - You're having a reaction to the anesthesia or the pain medication such as itching, nausea, or vomiting.
> - There's more heat, redness, or swelling around the incision than you might expect.
> - You have a sudden muscle ache, especially in your calf, that could indicate a life-threatening blood clot.

I'm a big believer in taking Vitamin C to promote healing. Increased doses of Vitamin C (2,000 mg per day) accelerate your recovery. You or your surgeon may have other ideas regarding diet and nutritional supplements that will best help you heal and stay healthy.

A week to two weeks after surgery, you'll return to your doctor to have the staples or sutures along your incision removed. I believe the skin is an indicator of how things are healing underneath. That's the art to medicine. I can look at a wound in my office and see that a patient has been on cortisone, or that he has an immune deficiency, is diabetic, or has poor circulation. The wound is my indicator, my litmus test for overall healing. Depending upon what I see at the incision site, I may decide to leave a patient in an immobilizer a bit longer to wait for further maturity of the wound. I keep watch over my postsurgical patients myself, because I can't go by a cookbook. I made the incision, I did the surgery, I sewed up the wound myself; now I want my experience and my judgment to help advise on the progress. Insist on having your own surgeon inspect the incision.

During this first office visit, seek approval to begin a pool program. (I'm comfortable letting my patients go into the pool about two weeks after surgery.) In the water, you'll be able to perform many safe movements that are still difficult on land. The sooner you start moving, the sooner you'll regain strength to make those same movements against gravity's force on land.

> **DRIVING AFTER SURGERY**
> How long before you can drive again depends on which knee had the surgery and on what kind of car you drive. If it was your left knee and the car you drive is not too low to the ground (a sports car) or too high (an SUV) and has an automatic shift, you'll be driving a lot sooner than if you had the operation on your right knee and you drive a sports car. It takes longer to feel comfortable driving a stick shift.

## RECOVERY TIMELINE

Every patient's recovery from surgery is unique in various ways, because every body is a little different. You may not respond exactly as another person did to surgery, and it's okay if you don't progress exactly down the same pathway. That doesn't mean something is wrong.

It's hard to give exact times, because much also depends on how you answer these questions: How is your general medical health? What is the condition of your other knee? Your back? Your hips? Have you had previous knee surgery? Here are some of the guidelines I suggest to my patients, but discuss your specific case with your surgeon.

### Meniscus Surgery (arthroscopy)

- STITCHES REMOVED. Sutures are removed one week later. You can now get into the pool (see Chapters 9 and 10.)
- ONE TO TWO WEEKS. You can generally play golf by now. As for other activities, you have no restrictions except pain. Back off any exercise that causes increased pain and switch to the nurturing activities of pool exercise, bicycling, and Nordic Track until you've been pain-free at least one week. (See Chapter 4 for nurturing exercise programs.)

- THREE MONTHS. When you wake up, you probably won't think of your knee as the first thought of the day. By now you're far away from the surgery in many ways. You're feeling quite good about being able to participate in your normal activities.
- ONE YEAR. Complete recovery. The scar tissue has evolved: it has healed, broken down, and healed again, finally making functional scar tissue that allows you to move well.

## ACL Surgery

- STITCHES REMOVED. This usually happens ten days to two weeks after surgery. As soon as the stitches or staples come out, you can get into the pool (see Chapters 9 and 10).
- SIX TO EIGHT WEEKS. Your surgeon will advise on when you can eliminate the brace. You can generally ride your outdoor bike by now and you probably don't need to be wearing the brace anymore. You still should avoid pivoting.
- THREE MONTHS. This is the end of your first major wall of recovery. You should be at the point where most of the pain from surgery is waning. You'll feel fewer snaps and pops from scar tissue. In fact, you may have a morning when you wake up and don't think of your knee as the first thought of the day. You can do most activitites at this point, but listen to your inner voice. If it tells you, "Stop! I'm nervous," you should stop. If it says, "I can do that," try it gently before diving all the way into the activity in question.
- SIX MONTHS. By now you're far away from the surgery in many ways. You're feeling quite good about being able to participate in your normal activities.
- ONE-YEAR ANNIVERSARY. In most cases, this is what your knee is going to be like from now on. There won't be many changes anymore. The scar tissue has evolved: it has healed, broken down, and healed again, finally making functional scar tissue that allows you to move well. You'll visit your doctor one year after surgery, then return only if you or your surgeon are concerned.

### Knee Implant Surgery

- STITCHES REMOVED. This usually happens ten days to two weeks after surgery. As soon as the stitches or staples come out, you can get into the pool (see Chapters 9 and 10).

- SIX TO EIGHT WEEKS. You can generally play golf by now, as long as you ride in a cart. Your knee will still be swollen and stiff, but you can be in the pool and on your bike. You can take walks around the block and you can go up and down stairs. You've reached the first milestone: ninety percent of the scar tissue you need is there, but it'll take another ten months to achieve the final ten percent and to have the immature scar become a fully mature, functioning scar. At six weeks, you're halfway to three months, which is the biggest hurdle.

- THREE MONTHS. This is the end of your first major wall of recovery. You should be at the point where most of the pains from surgery should be waning. You'll feel fewer snaps and pops from scar tissue. In fact, you may have a morning when you wake up and don't think of your knee as the first thought of the day. You can do most activitites at this point, but listen to your inner voice. If it tells you, "Stop! I'm nervous," you should stop. If it says, "I can do that," try it gently before diving all the way into the activity in question.

- SIX MONTHS. By now you're far away from the surgery in many ways. You're feeling quite good about being able to participate in your normal activities. You may still have some stiffness, but be patient and continue with your rehabilitation exercises.

- ONE-YEAR ANNIVERSARY. In most cases, this is what your knee is going to be like from now on. There won't be many more changes. The scar tissue has evolved: it has healed, broken down, healed again, finally making functional scar tissue that allows you to move well.

- LIFETIME. Your new knee needs to be watched, even when it's working well for you. Your surgeon will most likely want you to come for regular checkups every year, so he or she can take an X ray to evaluate the status of your knee. Has the plastic begun to wear? Has the prosthesis begun to loosen from the bone? These are "silent findings," meaning you won't have any symptoms to alert you to these problems, so you should see your surgeon every year.

---

**VISIT YOUR SURGEON EVERY YEAR AFTER KNEE IMPLANT SURGERY**

A man who'd had total knee surgery on both knees came to me ten years later because one of his knees was bothering him. His previous surgeon didn't follow him, and he didn't have X rays during those ten years. When I took an X ray, I found that he had worn through the plastic completely, had broken the titanium component in his tibia, and had also broken the bone beneath it. If he'd been followed annually with an X ray, his doctor would have seen the wear and taken him back to surgery for an easy replacement of the plastic. Instead, I had to remove the implants, work on his fractured tibia, then replace the implants and the plastic. He'd had no symptoms and no pain until it was too late.

---

Just how long any implant will last depends on the bone, the implant, and the patient. Over ninety percent of the patients with knee implants are still doing well fifteen and twenty years later, and we expect some of the newer implants we're using to last up to thirty years.

# 14 AFTER SURGERY

*With Tanya Moran-Dougherty, MPT*

Memory can be your worst enemy in the weeks and months following surgery. You remember how far you used to run or walk, how many sets of tennis you used to play, how many golf courses you used to visit each year. You will probably find that "used to" phrase in both your thoughts and your conversations. But as basketball legend Wilt Chamberlain always said, "Old Man 'Used To' is dead and gone."

What you used to do no longer applies. Forget it, and start with where you are right now.

Your postsurgical knee requires planning, pampering, and patience. You need to plan your recovery with care, pamper your aching knee that sometimes won't feel as if it belongs to you, and have patience knowing that the human body heals: that's what it is innately programmed to do. "Tincture of Time" plus ice and the proper exercises will help you regain your strength and flexibility, allowing you once again to be mobile and comfortable as you move through your daily life and recreational activities.

You may have become familiar with all the exercises in the pool and land therapy programs of Chapters 10 and 11 as you tried to prevent knee surgery. Your efforts may have turned into prehab; that is, rehabilitation prior to surgery. In that case, you entered the operating room well-prepared for the ordeals of surgery. Or you may have found this book only after you had knee surgery and you now wish to use our pool and land programs to speed your recovery. This chapter will guide you through the exercises at the right pace so you don't disrupt the healing process.

---

**ICE, ICE, AND MORE ICE**

Ice your knee in the morning, the afternoon, and the evening. Keep icing for a week after surgery. Keep icing a month after surgery. Keep icing your knee at the first sign of pain, inflammation, or swelling. Consider ice your primary pain-killing medicine.

---

## THE THREE PHASES OF POSTSURGICAL REHABILITATION

### Phase One

Right after surgery, you will find yourself in the first phase of rehabilitation, which is characterized by the following:

PAIN. You'll have nearly constant, moderate to severe pain on a daily basis. Pain is caused by inflammation. You may even begin to notice increased pain in your "good" knee from the greater work its doing.

INFLAMMATION. Traumatized tissues release chemical irritants that stimulate nerve impulses, creating the pain experience and relaying that pain. Inflammation also causes swelling.

SWELLING (EDEMA). Swelling is the body's natural response to trauma in order to immobilize the area. Swelling causes increased pain as it puts pressure on the nerves. Further, swelling causes a loss of mobility.

LOSS OF MOBILITY. Swelling causes increased pressure

within your knee joint and the surrounding tissues, which makes it difficult to move your knee. The pain you feel stimulates "splinting," or increased muscular contraction in the area to protect your knee.

LOSS OF FUNCTION. When mobility is lost in your knee, you will also lose function. When the muscles are in "splinting" mode, your knee can quickly become stiff.

RAPID LOSS OF FITNESS LEVEL. Without mobility or function, you lose fitness. Unless you quickly begin rehabilitation exercises, your overall body fitness will quickly decline.

---

### UP WITH THE GOOD; DOWN WITH THE BAD

A standard refrain among patients who have recently had surgery on their knees is "Up with the good; down with the bad." It's an easy slogan to remember whenever you want to step onto a curb or stair. You want to step **up with your good knee first.** Conversely, when going down a stair or curb, you want to step **down first with your postsurgical knee.** You'll know you're getting better when you can go up or down with either leg first.

---

The goals of Phase One are to resolve all of the previously mentioned issues, but the major emphasis is on eliminating pain, inflammation, and swelling. All six of these factors are easily addressed in the pool. The cooling effect of the water helps decrease pain and inflammation while the hydrostatic pressure the water exerts on your knee helps push out swelling. You will be able to move much sooner and more easily in water than you could on land, so begin your postsurgical rehab in the pool. Of course, your incision site must be healed enough to prevent infection.

You'll begin your land exercises right away as well. Let pain be your guide. If an exercise increases your knee pain, stop. Skip it and try the next exercise. If the land exercises seem too difficult or painful at first, spend your first week in the pool. If you don't have access to a pool, you'll be focusing on the land exercises.

Most postsurgical knee patients will begin gentle weightbearing as early as possible in Phase One. You may need a knee brace, a cane, crutches, or a walker, but you'll want to begin normalizing your gait right away. Don't hesitate to use these devices. They are an important part of your recovery. Your surgeon will give you any restrictions about weightbearing.

## Phase Two

You enter Phase Two when you can identify your first significant reduction of symptoms. This means you notice that you have less pain and swelling as well as improved mobility and function. Phase Two is characterized by minimal to moderate intermittent pain that comes from movement, such as the activities of daily living. Although symptoms have begun to decrease, moderate inflammation and swelling are still present, and a moderate loss of mobility and function still exists. It is time to begin regaining strength and flexibility to prepare for the more strenuous rehabilitation to follow. You can expect to feel some moderate pain when you move your knee, but (except for total knee patients) don't force an exercise and increase your pain beyond that moderate level.

The goals of Phase Two continue to be the reduction of pain, inflammation, and swelling; however, the major emphasis turns to increasing your flexibility and strength so you can return to normal walking and weightbearing.

> **A WEIGHTBEARING TEST**
> Can you perform a single-leg stance on your healing leg for three to five seconds without pain and without feeling instability in your knee? If so, you can progress to land weightbearing Exercises 12 to 15. If you feel even a twinge of pain, or if your knee feels vulnerable or at all unstable, stick with non-weightbearing Exercises 1 to 11 on land and try to increase your squats and step work in the pool. In that way, you'll generate increased strength in and around your knee that will soon begin to translate into improved function on land.

## Phase Three

Phase Three begins when you can accomplish basic ADLs with ease and can tolerate functional weightbearing exercises to some degree. You may not have mastered higher-level activities such as reciprocal stair climbing, squatting without using your upper body, or recreational sports and activities. By this time you should be experiencing only minimal intermittent pain that occurs solely during activity. Inflammation and swelling should be minimal as well. It is during Phase Three that many people stop short of their goals of full recovery. The almost imperceptible swelling, chronic inflammation, incomplete range of motion, and decrease in strength, are the last traces of your surgery, and they are very real obstacles to regaining full function.

Keep going with your pool and land rehabilitation exercises until you reach the goals of Phase Three, to be relatively painfree with few or no symptoms. Ultimately, you want no pain and no symptoms; those goals may take up to a year to accomplish. The better the long-range function you expect from your knee, the longer you will need to continue with your rehabilitation.

**REMAIN CAUTIOUS AND DELIBERATE**

Somewhere in the middle of a rehab session, you're going to have the thought, "I could go back to playing tennis—today!" **Don't.** If you retain your caution and deliberateness throughout this period, your progress will generally be steady and consistent. If you overdo things now and then, an occasional setback—pain, swelling, undue soreness—may require extra days in the pool away from gravity. Don't get upset; just do the work. It's all part of the normal comeback for athletes and nonathletes alike. But then, vow not to make the same mistake again that triggered the setback. By taking charge of your knee and assuming full responsibility for any risks you take with it, you can earn a knee that serves you beautifully for a lifetime.

Phase Three is a good time to review your biomechanics. Focus on changing any incorrect movement patterns in your ADLs and fitness activities that may have contributed to the deterioration of your knee.

**TIPS FOR POSTSURGICAL SESSIONS**

**ICE AFTER EACH SESSION.** Ice can make the difference between recovering from a session or not. If you ice, you may not be sore, stiff, or have as much pain tomorrow.

**DON'T TRY TO DO TOO MUCH.** If pain and swelling increase after a session and persist after icing, you've worked too hard. If swelling and stiffness persist for more than twenty-four hours, reduce your workout intensity by moving more slowly and doing fewer repetitions.

**DO *ONLY* THE PHASE ONE EXERCISES WHEN YOU ARE IN PHASE ONE.** Do only Phase Two exercises while in Phase Two, and so on.

If you had meniscus surgery, continue reading the next section, where you'll find your three phases of rehabilitation. If you had ACL surgery, follow the program that begins on page 274. If you had knee implant surgery, turn to page 282. Others who don't fall cleanly into one of these categories can also use the programs. Those who have had a surgical repair of a fracture should follow the ACL protocol, while those who have sprained their knees should ask their doctors if they had a Grade 1, 2, or 3 ligament injury. Grades 1 and 2 (partial ligament tear) should follow the meniscus program; Grade 3 (a complete ligament tear) should follow the ACL program.

## MENISCUS OR OTHER ARTHROSCOPIC SURGERY

Arthroscopic surgeries are considered minimally-invasive procedures. No major incisions were made and little work was performed inside the joint, so you'll be fairly mobile and able to do a lot more than other types of knee-surgery patients. You might even be able to go up and down stairs fairly quickly after surgery.

### Phase One.

If you have access to a pool, start there, then try the land program two days later. Skip a day between sessions your first week and concentrate on icing and elevating your leg. Do one pool then one land session every other day. (If you feel an increase in your pain, inflammation, and swelling after the land session, stick with the pool for your first post-op week.)

**Begin slowly, move gently, and proceed with caution.** If you feel increased pain, narrow your range of motion or move even more slowly. Follow this Phase One program until your symptoms begin to subside.

## POOL:

During your first day in the pool, if you find yourself not wanting to bend your postsurgical knee, you can start with a straight-leg program for the first week or two. (See page 161 for a straight-leg pool program.)  To protect your healing knee from impact, you'll want to do the non-weightbearing deep-water exercises, so even if you're a nonswimmer, put on a flotation belt and hold onto the side of the pool. (See pages 150 to 151 for help in selecting the correct flotation for your body type.) When you do the knee-bending exercises, start slowly and gently. **Use care when doing the heel lifts (Exercise 6) and hamstring curls (Exercise 31).** If you feel pain doing those exercises, limit the range of the motion until your knee has had more time to heal. If you don't have pain, but your knee doesn't want to bend very far, push it gently so you can achieve the range of motion you need.

- DEEP-WATER INTERVALS: low-intensity level          15 minutes
  Consider a straight-leg program for a few weeks (see page 161).
      (See Exercises 1 to 4, pages 158 to 165.)
- DEEP WATERPOWER: sit kicks, heel lifts          20 reps each
      (See Exercises 5 and 6, pages 165 to 166.)
- KICK TRAINING: all          30 seconds each
      (See Exercises 8 to 11, pages 168 to 171.)
- GAIT TRAINING: walking forward, backward, sideways   1 minute each
      (See Exercise 12, pages 173 to 174.)
- STRETCHING: curl and stretch, hamstring stretch,
  body swing, quad stretch          30 seconds each
      (See Exercises 15 to 18, pages 177 to 179.)
- LOWER EXTREMITY EXERCISES: lateral leg raises, standing
  leg swings, quad extensions, hamstring curls          15 reps each
      (See Exercises 28 to 31, pages 189 to 192.)

## LAND:

During your first week after surgery, perform the non-weight-bearing exercises only (Exercises 1 to 11). Stay within your painfree range of motion, which is especially important while you're healing after surgery. Bend your knee only to the point where you feel some discomfort. Do not create more pain. Begin with one set of ten reps for each of the non-weightbearing exercises and, of course, ice after each session with your leg elevated. Because this surgery is minimally-invasive, you will begin the weightbearing exercises during your second week in Phase One. You may be surprised how easily you will be walking in just a week. By starting these land exercises right away, you'll strengthen the muscles needed to perform your daily functional activities.

If you don't have access to a pool, which serves as your primary fitness activity in a pool/land combined program, a stationary or recumbent bicycle is a safe alternative. Position your seat so your knee bends comfortably at 90 to 100 degrees. If you allow your knee to bend more than that, you could irritate your patella during deep bending on the upstroke, plus you won't have your seat high enough for full extension on the downstroke.

- NON-WEIGHTBEARING EXERCISES: all
  (See Exercises 1 and 5 to 11 on pages 202,     10 reps
  203, and 208 to 212.)
  hamstring stretch, quad stretch, gastroc stretch     3 x 30 seconds
  (See Exercises 2 to 4 on pages 203 to 206.)

- WEIGHTBEARING EXERCISES: all          10 reps each
  (See Exercises 12 to 15, pages 213 to 214.)

- BICYCLING: stationary or recumbent bike          5 to 10 minutes,
                                                   0 resistance

## Phase Two

Your pain, inflammation, and swelling are coming down now, so it's time to increase your workload by adding more exercises, more sets, and more reps. Continue to let pain be your guide and adjust your program if needed. You can always go back to Phase One for a week if that seems like the right thing for your knee.

### POOL:

You'll be adding your first exercises that call for impact in the shallow end of the pool, so notice that you **must** wear a flotation belt in this phase. The belt allows you to jump upward, creating power and strength in your knee, but the belt and the water—not your knee—will catch you as you land. You'll continue wearing the belt as you begin shallow-water running.

- DEEP-WATER INTERVALS: medium-intensity level        20 minutes
  (See Exercises 1 to 4, pages 158 to 165.)
- DEEP WATERPOWER: all        30 reps each
  (See Exercises 5 to 7, pages 165 to 167.)
- KICK TRAINING: all        45 seconds each
  (See Exercises 8 to 11, pages 168 to 171.)
- GAIT TRAINING: all        1 minute each
  (See Exercises 12 to 14, pages 173 to 176.
  Wear a float belt during bouncing, Exercise 14.)
- WATERPOWER WORKOUT EXERCISES:        10 reps **with belt**
  lunges, squat jumps, power frog jumps,
  (See Exercises 21, 22, and 25, pages 181, 182 and 184.)
  running with belt, low-intensity program   2 to 6 minutes
  (See Exercise 27, pages 185 to 186.)
- STRETCHING: all        30 seconds each
  (See Exercises 15 to 20, pages 177 to 180.)
- LOWER EXTREMITY EXERCISES: all        30 reps each
  (See Exercises 28 to 34, pages 189 to 195.)

## LAND:

Increase your number of non-weightbearing repetitions to two sets of ten reps, or twenty reps total. If you're able to stand on your surgical leg for three to five seconds without any buckling or instability, you'll also add functional exercises and the easiest resistance exercise in Phase Two. When you do Exercise 22, begin with the easiest (yellow) Thera-band. Increase to a stronger Thera-Band each session if you can comfortably perform your repetitions. If you feel fatigue after ten reps, stay with that color Thera-Band until those ten reps become easy.

- NON-WEIGHTBEARING EXERCISES: all
    (See Exercises 1 and 5 to 11 on pages 202,     2 x 10 reps
     203, and 208 to 212.)
    hamstring stretch, quad stretch, gastroc stretch     3 x 30 seconds
    (See Exercises 2 to 4 on pages 203 to 206.)

- WEIGHTBEARING EXERCISES: all     2 sets of 10 reps each
    (See Exercises 12 to 15, pages 213 to 214.)

- FUNCTIONAL EXERCISES: wall slides, good mornings,     10 reps each
    step ups, side step ups, mini squats
    (See Exercises 16 to 19 and Exercise 21 on
     pages 214 to 218.)

- RESISTANCE EXERCISES: terminal extension
    with Thera-Band, quad extension with Thera-Band,     10 reps
    hamstring curls with Thera-Band
    (See Exercises 22 to 24 on pages 219 to 220.)

- BICYCLING: stationary or recumbent bike     10 to 20 minutes,
         0 resistance

## Phase Three

Now you're ready for increased impact in the pool and more functional exercises on land, but you must add those exercises gradually. In Phase Two you did the four safest Waterpower Workout exercises while wearing a flotation belt. You jumped upward using your muscular strength, but the belt, not your knee, caught most of your weight as you landed. Now, at the beginning of Phase Three, wear a belt until you've mastered all six of the Waterpower jumping exercises and can do thirty reps of each. Then it's time to remove your belt and start over with twenty reps of each exercise. You'll be surprised how much harder the exercises are without your belt, so don't try for too many reps too quickly. Similarly, when you add the resistance boot to your lower extremity exercises, you'll feel how much harder the exercise is, so drop your reps to twenty and work your way back up to thirty reps gradually. This may seem slow, but it's your surest way to progress without re-injury.

In your land program, you'll increase your reps by one set. At the beginning of Phase Three, you'll start doing two sets of functional and resistance exercises, 16 to 25, and you'll progress to three sets of ten reps by the end of Phase Three. Begin Phase Three with the Thera-Band color that allows you to perform comfortably eight repetitions but you feel fatigue after ten reps. Progress to a Thera-Band with more resistance as indicated in the table on page 219.

### POOL:

- DEEP-WATER INTERVALS: high-intensity level                25 minutes
    (See Exercises 1 to 4, pages 158 to 165.)
- DEEP WATERPOWER: all                                              50 reps each
    (See Exercises 5 to 7, pages 165 to 167.)

- KICK TRAINING: all                         1 minute each
    (See Exercises 8 to 11, pages 168 to 171.
    Work harder the last 30 seconds.)
- GAIT TRAINING: all (no belt)           1 minute each
    (See Exercises 12 to 14, pages 173 to 176.)
- WATERPOWER WORKOUT EXERCISES: all (no belt)    20 to 30 reps
    (See Exercises 21 to 26, pages 181 to 184.
    When belt removed, start at twenty reps again and
    work up to thirty.)
    running, no belt, high-intensity program      11 minutes
    (See Exercise 27, page 185 to 187.)
- STRETCHING: all                     30 seconds each
    See Exercises 15 to 20, pages 177 to 180.)
- LOWER EXTREMITY EXERCISES: all        30 reps each
    Add boot, start at twenty reps again and work up to thirty.
    (See Exercises 28 to 34, pages 189 to 195.)

## LAND:

- NON-WEIGHTBEARING EXERCISES: all
    (See Exercises 1 and 5 to 11 on pages     3 x 10 reps
    202, 203, and 208 to 212.)
    hamstring stretch, quad stretch, gastroc stretch    3 x 30 seconds
    (See Exercises 2 to 4 on pages 203 to 206.)

- WEIGHTBEARING EXERCISES: all      3 sets of 10 reps each
    (See Exercises 12 to15, pages 213 to 214.)

- FUNCTIONAL EXERCISES: all       2-3 sets of 10 reps each
    (See Exercises 16 to 21 on pages 214 to 218.)

- RESISTANCE EXERCISES: all       2-3 sets of 10 reps each
    (See Exercises 22 to 25 on pages 219 to 221
    and the table on page 219.)

- BICYCLING: stationary or recumbent bike    20 to 30 minutes with
    minimum tension

## ANTERIOR CRUCIATE LIGAMENT SURGERY

Your primary concern after ACL surgery is to protect the repair site where the new ligament was attached inside your knee. To do that, **you must not straighten your knee *against resistance or a weight* for six weeks.** If you extend your knee against resistance, you apply direct pressure onto your vulnerable surgical site and could potentially tear your graft. This means you won't be doing quad extensions with an ankle weight at home or using a quad machine at the gym. It means you won't be kicking a ball, reaching to hold open a door with your foot, or quickly kicking the covers off your legs when rising from bed. By contrast, straightening your leg in the pool or on land **without resistance or a weight** will be recommended.

Strengthening your hamstring muscles **against resistance** is fine—resistance work on those muscles won't hurt your graft. In fact, the stronger your hamstring muscles are, the more protection you have for your new ACL. That's because the hamstring muscles attach in a position that protects your knee in much the same way your ACL does. Both the ACL and the hamstrings hold the tibia in place against forces that would otherwise cause that lower-leg bone to move forward.

Begin Phase One exercises slowly, move gently, and proceed with caution. If you feel increased pain, narrow your range of motion or move even more slowly. Follow this Phase One program until your symptoms begin to subside.

### Phase One

Now that your knee has been stabilized with a newly reconstructed ACL, you may be thinking that you're free to use your knee as normally as possible. However, for now, you need to practice caution with all activities. In particular, you need to avoid twisting and pivoting motions on a planted foot. During the first six weeks of your recovery, it's critical that you do not disrupt healing with dangerous movements but do everything in your power to ensure the surgeon's work will be protected as it heals.

All of the ligaments that stabilize and support your knee also provide feedback to your body regarding where your knee is in space and in relationship to other joints. This invisible perception is called your kinesthetic sense. For example, when you're standing on one leg to put your pants on, you naturally know where to move your weight in order to balance and avoid falling. Without kinesthetic sense, you would have no idea how to balance on one leg. After surgery, you will experience a loss of this kinesthetic sense due to swelling, disruption of the muscles, and numbness around your incision site. Your knee will be unstable due to the combination of decreased kinesthetic sense and decreased strength. It takes time for you to regain your confidence in all of your abilities. (You may find that watching yourself in a mirror as you perform your ADLs will give you good feedback.)

To improve your kinesthetic sense and move toward full rehabilitation, you must do the following:

- **CONTROL SWELLING.** Ice and elevate your knee for ten to fififteen minutes at least three to four times a day. Excessive swelling inside the joint after ACL surgery will cause a phenomenon known as "quad shut-down." This is the body's protective mechanism to keep you from putting too much weight on your knee.
- **STRENGTHEN YOUR QUADRICEPS MUSCLES.** To counteract "quad shut-down," do two to three quad sets (Exercise 5, page 208) a day as shown in the land program that follows. The Phase One exercises in the pool and on land challenge your quads in various ways to accelerate the strengthening process, but you need to assume full responsibility for getting your quads working again by making sure you do your quad sets.

- **INITIATE EARLY AND CONTROLLED WEIGHTBEARING.** Weight-bearing exercises stimulate receptors in the joints, muscles, and ligaments to provide you with additional kinesthetic information. Further, weightbearing creates a co-contraction of the muscles surrounding your knee—a simultaneous contraction of the quads, hamstrings, and gastrocs that enhances joint stability. You'll be able to begin weightbearing in the pool long before such movements might be feasible on land. Keep in mind, however, that even in the pool you must avoid twisting and pivoting on a planted foot. On land, do not begin weightbearing on your postsurgical knee until you can pass the weightbearing test on page 265.

---

**REACH FOR FULL EXTENSION QUICKLY**
The latest research shows that patients who reach full extension soon after ACL surgery have less patellofemoral pain then those patients who have limited extension. This means you should do knee extensions right away in the pool without a resistance device and on land you should do them slowly against gravity but *without a weight* **until at least six weeks after surgery.**

---

One of the most important goals for this phase is to restore full extension in your knee as soon as possible while protecting the graft. Without full extension, you'll be walking around on a partially bent knee, which aggravates the patella and causes patellofemoral pain. To reach full extension, you should avoid sleeping with a pillow under your knee even though you may find that comforting. Don't force your knee into full extension, but try this: ice your knee with the leg straight in front of you. The weight of the ice combined with gravity will help stretch your knee to full extension. Follow the program below with great care in order to protect your healing graft, and, of course, ice after each session with your leg elevated.

If you don't have access to a pool, which serves as your primary fitness activity in a pool/land combined program, a stationary or recumbent bicycle is a safe alternative. It's a great way to improve your knee ROM and to strengthen your quadriceps. However, since your surgeon has the most knowledge regarding the strength of your graft, ask him or her for guidelines before bicycling for exercise. If your doctor says okay, position the seat so your knee comfortably bends to 90 to 100 degrees. If you allow your knee to bend more than that, you could irritate your patella during deep bending on the upstroke, plus you won't have your seat high enough for full extension on the downstroke. If you're wearing a knee brace, check with your surgeon to see if you can remove it for bicycling.

## POOL:

- DEEP-WATER INTERVALS: low-intensity level — 15 minutes
  (See Exercises 1 to 4, pages 158 to 163.)
- DEEP WATERPOWER: sit kicks, heel lifts — 20 reps each
  (See Exercises 5 and 6, pages 165 to 166.)
- KICK TRAINING: all — 30 seconds each
  (See Exercises 8 to 11, pages 168 to 171.)
- GAIT TRAINING: walking forward, backward, sideways — 1 minute each
  (See Exercise 12, pages 173 to 174.)
- STRETCHING: curl and stretch, hamstring stretch, — 30 seconds each
  body swing, gastroc stretch
  (See Exercises 15 to 17, and Exercise 20,
  pages 177 to 178 and page 180.)
- LOWER EXTREMITY EXERCISES: lateral leg raises,
  standing leg swings, quad extensions, hamstring — 15 reps each
  curls, squats, heel/toe raises
  (See Exercises 28 to 33, pages 189 to 193.)

## LAND:

- NON-WEIGHTBEARING EXERCISES: heel slides          10 reps
    (See Exercise 1 on pages 202 to 203.)
  hamstring stretch, gastroc stretch          3 x 30 seconds
                                              (2 to 3 times/day)
    (See Exercises 2 and 4 on pages 203 and 206.)
  quad sets, hamstring sets,          10 reps each
                                      (2 to 3 times/day)

    (See Exercises 5 and 6 on page 208.)
  straight leg raises, hip abduction,          10 reps each
  hip adduction, hip extension, quad extensions
    (See Exercises 7 to 11 on pages 209 to 212.)
- WEIGHTBEARING EXERCISES:
  hamstring curls          10 reps (on
                           surgical knee only)

    (See Exercise 12 on page 213.)
- Stationary or recumbent bike          5 to 10 minutes,
                                        0 resistance

  Adjust the seat higher (upright bike) or farther back
  (recumbent bike) to accommodate your knee's range of movement.

## Phase Two

Even if your insurance doesn't cover it, this is the time when you probably should pay for some visits to a physical therapist to receive skilled guidance in setting up your plan. Recovery from ACL surgery is tricky, and you don't want to be too aggressive or too cautious as you try to regain your full mobility.

---

**FOUR-WEEK WARNING**

Your ACL graft is at its weakest between four and six weeks after surgery—even more so than immediately after the operation. During that time your new ACL is developing its blood supply and is very vulnerable. Don't disrupt its healing by becoming careless a month after surgery.

---

## POOL:

You'll be in that dangerous four- to six-week period as you enter Phase Two. This means you must be cautious, even in the pool. Don't plant your foot and make any pivoting movements when turning during gait training Exercises 12 and 13. Don't twist your knee doing the quad stretch Exercise 18, and **wear a flotation belt until six weeks after surgery when you do Waterpower Workout Exercises 21 to 27.**

At the beginning of Phase Two, you'll start doing twenty reps of the step work and build to thirty reps by the time you've completed Phase Two. Since you can't do this movement easily on land, it's vital that you gain both skill and strength in step work in the pool. Once you can do thirty pool stepovers, you'll feel more confident doing step work on land.

* DEEP-WATER INTERVALS: medium-intensity level     20 minutes
    (See Exercises 1 to 4, pages 158 to 163.)
* DEEP WATERPOWER: all     30 reps each
    (See Exercises 5 to 7, pages 165 to 167.)
* KICK TRAINING: all     45 seconds each
    (See Exercises 8 to 11, pages 168 to 171.)
* GAIT TRAINING: walking forward, backward,     1 minute each
    sideways, marching
    (See Exercises 12 and 13, pages 173 to 175.)
* WATERPOWER WORKOUT EXERCISES:     10 reps (**with belt**)
    lunges, squat jumps, power frog jumps,
    (See Exercises 21, 22, and 25, pages 181, 182 and 184.)
    running **with belt**, low-intensity program     4 to 6 minutes
    (See Exercise 27, pages 185 to 186. After six weeks,
    move to medium-intensity program 4 to 8 minutes.)
* STRETCHING: all     30 seconds each
    (See Exercises 15 to 20, pages 177 to 180.
    Use a strap and extreme care doing the quad stretch and hip
    flexor stretch, Exercises 18 and 19. Do not twist your knee.)

- LOWER EXTREMITY EXERCISES:  all                                  20 to 30 reps each
    (See Exercises 28 to 34, pages 189 to 195.
    Start with twenty reps of each, build to thirty.)

## LAND:

During Phase Two, you will begin more weightbearing  and
functional exercises on land. Do your best to tolerate these exercises as much as you can—the sooner you do weightbearing
well, the sooner you'll be walking and moving normally. As
you attempt early weightbearing, be aware of the improvements
you make in both your kinesthetic sense and your overall leg
strength. This phase is critical in the healing process: you need
to balance the increase in your weightbearing and functional
activities with extreme care in protecting your graft by avoiding
pivoting and twisting movements. You still should not be performing any resistive exercises for your quadriceps such as leg
extensions with weights or on knee machines.

By now you should have full extension in your knee. If you
don't, add more hamstring and gastroc stretches both in the
pool and on land. In the pool, add a flotation cuff to your quad
extensions, Exercise 30. If you've been wearing a brace, your
surgeon will advise you when you can remove it. (Typically,
you'll be braced for at least four to six weeks.)

- NON-WEIGHTBEARING EXERCISES: heel slides        2 x 10 reps
    (See Exercise 1 on pages 202 to 203.)

    hamstring stretch, gastroc stretch        3 x 30 seconds
                                              (2 to 3 times/day)
        (See Exercises 2 and 4 on pages 203 and 206.)

    quad stretch        3 x 30 seconds
        (See Exercise 3 on page 204. Be extremely careful
        when doing this stretch. Do not twist your knee.)

    quad sets, hamstring sets        2 x 10 reps each
    straight leg raises, hip abduction,        2 x 10 reps each
    hip adduction, hip extension, quad extensions
        (See Exercises 5 to 11 on pages 208 to 212.)

- WEIGHTBEARING EXERCISES: hamstring curls       2 x 10 reps each
  toe raises, single leg stance
      (See Exercises 12 to 14 on page 213.)
- FUNCTIONAL EXERCISES: wall slides, step-ups,      10 reps each
  mini-squats
      (See Exercises 16, 18, and 21 on pages 214 to 216,
      and 218. Stay in a painfree range of movement during
      wall slides. Use a four-inch step on step-ups.)
- RESISTANCE EXERCISES: terminal extension with
  Thera-Band                                      10 reps
      (See Exercise 22 on page 219.)
- BICYCLING: stationary or recumbent bike,      10 to 20 minutes,
                                                         0 resistance
  Adjust the seat higher (upright bike) or farther back (recumbent bike)
  to accommodate your knee's range of movement.

## Phase Three

By now you're safely past the dangerous four- to six-week period when your healing graft is most vulnerable. You should be accomplishing your activities of daily living fairly easily and tolerating weightbearing on your postsurgical knee to some degree. Now, to aim toward full recovery, you must further increase your leg strength and weightbearing capacity. To do this, you'll remove your flotation belt in the pool, add the hardest of the land exercises, and progress to a Thera-Band of stronger resistance.

## Pool:

- DEEP-WATER INTERVALS: high-intensity level      25 minutes
      (See Exercises 1 to 4, pages 158 to 165.)
- DEEP WATERPOWER: all                          50 reps each
      (See Exercises 5 to 7, pages 165 to 167.)
- KICK TRAINING: all                         1 minute each
      (See Exercises 8 to 11, pages 168 to 171.
      Increase speed the last thirty seconds.)

- GAIT TRAINING: all                                            1 minute each
    (See Exercises 12 to 14, pages 173 to 176.)
- STRETCHING: all                                               30 seconds each
    (See Exercises 15 to 20, pages 177 to 180.)
- WATERPOWER WORKOUT EXERCISES: all, no belt                    20 to 30 reps
    (See Exercises 21 to 26, pages 181 to 184)
    running, no belt, high intensity program                   6 minutes
    (See Exercise 27, pages 185 to 187.)
- LOWER EXTREMITY EXERCISES: all                                20 to 30 reps each
    (See Exercises 28 to 34, pages 189 to 195.
    Start with twenty reps of each, build to thirty reps.)

## LAND:

- NON-WEIGHTBEARING EXERCISES: all
    (See Exercises 1 and 5 to 11 on pages 202,     3 x 10 reps
      203, and 208 to 212.)
    hamstring stretch, quad stretch, gastroc stretch    3 x 30 seconds
    (See Exercises 2 to 4 on pages 203 to 206.)
- WEIGHTBEARING EXERCISES: all                        2 to 3 x 10 reps each
    (See Exercises 12 to15 on pages 213 to 214.)
- FUNCTIONAL EXERCISES: all                            2 to 3 x 10 reps
    (See Exercises 16 to 21 on pages 214 to 218. Try
    to reach 90 degrees on wall slides and single leg
    wall slides, and use a six-inch step on step work.)
- RESISTANCE EXERCISES: all
    (See Exercises 22 to 25 on pages 219 to 221.) 2 to 3 x 10 reps
- BICYCLING: stationary or recumbent bike             20 to 30 minutes,
                                                      minimal resistance
    Adjust the seat higher (upright bike) or farther back
    (recumbent bike) to accommodate your knee range of movement.

## KNEE IMPLANT SURGERY

Take your pain medications and fasten your seat belt, because you're the one postsurgical patient who needs to push. The race is on—you have less than six months to regain your flexion and extension. After that it's too late! Whatever knee movement you have at that time is all you can ever expect. That's why you'll push through discomfort and even push through pain in order to develop a knee that really works for the rest of your life.

## Phase One

Your knee implant is strong and secure, so there's no worry about tearing anything loose inside your knee. You'll have swelling for at least three months, and you may experience pain up to a year after surgery, but even while you're swollen and in pain, you need to work hard to regain enough flexion and extension in your knee to do all your normal ADLs. Focus first on getting full knee extension— you need to be able to fully straighten your knee in order to walk. Then work on gaining the maximum flexion possible. While you can expect soreness, swelling, and heat, be aware of any sudden changes in the appearance of your incision. (See page 254 regarding postsurgical emergencies.)

## POOL:

Consider your first week the honeymoon stage. If you have access to a pool, you'll do only the painfree exercises in the pool program. That means if an exercise hurts, you can skip it. This first week is the only time you don't have to face pain squarely and stare it down. After that, find your courage to do the work that will make your surgery pay off. During your first week, you can do less time and fewer reps than what is listed. By the second week, however, start doing all the exercises. If you experience sharp, shooting pain, slow the movement or narrow the range of motion. But if your knee is just stiff, swollen, and feels filled with fluid, try to work through that feeling. The pool exercises will help improve your circulation and the hydrostatic pressure helps push out the fluids of swelling. The quad stretch will be hard for you to do, so use a strap, or **you can duplicate the chair version of the land quad stretch (see photo 11-3B on page 205) by placing your foot on one of the pool's steps.**

- DEEP-WATER INTERVALS: low-intensity level      15 minutes
  (See Exercises 1 to 4, pages 158 to 163.)
- DEEP WATERPOWER: sit kicks, heel lifts      20 reps each
  (See Exercises 5 and 6, pages 165 to 166.)
- KICK TRAINING: all      30 seconds each
  (See Exercises 8 to 11, pages 168 to 171.)
- GAIT TRAINING: walking forward, backward, sideways
  marching      1 minute each
  (See Exercises 12 and 13, pages 173 to 175.)
- STRETCHING: curl and stretch, hamstring stretch,
  body swing      30 seconds each
  (See Exercises 15 to 17, pages 177 to 178.)
  quad stretch with strap or on step      3 x 30 seconds
  (See Exercise 18 on page 179 and Exercise 3B
  on page 205 on pool step.)
- LOWER EXTREMITY EXERCISES: lateral leg raises,
  standing leg swings, quad extensions, hamstring
  curls, squats, heel/toe raises      15 reps each
  (See Exercises 28 to 33, pages 189 to 193.)

## LAND:

You'll start your land program the second week in order to begin regaining strength in your movements against gravity. You have a limited window of opportunity to restore your range of motion, so get moving! While it's normal to have pain, don't let pain stop you from bending and straightening your knee as much as you can tolerate. Quad stretches are typically very difficult to perform in Phase One because of pain and significant limitations in range of movement, so you'll skip the quad stretch on land until Phase Two. When you do Exercise 12, hamstring curls, stand on your stronger leg and work **the surgical leg only**. If you're bicycling, you may not yet be able to complete one full revolution of the pedals because of limitations in your knee's range of motion. In that case, pedal backward and forward, each stroke attempting to bend your knee into more and more flexion.

- NON-WEIGHTBEARING EXERCISES: heel slides     I to 2 sets of 10 per day
  (See Exercise 1, pages 202 and 203.)
  hamstring stretch, gastroc stretch     3 x 30 seconds each
  (See Exercises 2 and 4, pages 203 and 206.)
  quad sets, hamstring sets, straight leg raises,     10 reps each
  hip abduction, hip adduction, hip extension, quad extension
  (See Exercises 5 to 11, pages 208 to 212.)
- WEIGHTBEARING EXERCISES: hamstring curls     10 reps
  (surgical leg only)
  (See Exercise 12, page 213.)
- RESISTANCE EXERCISES: terminal knee extensions     10 reps
  with Thera-band
  (See Exercise 22, page 219.)
- BICYCLING: stationary or recumbent bike     5 to 10 minutes, 0 tension

## Phase Two

In Phase Two your pain won't be as constant or as intense. Your range of motion will begin to improve so you'll be able to perform your ADLs more easily. It won't be as difficult to rise from a toilet or chair, your knee won't feel as stiff when walking, and you may be able to climb stairs leading with your surgical leg. If you're bicycling, you should be able to complete a full revolution during this phase. Descending stairs will still be difficult, but don't worry—that's normal. You'll keep getting better at it, especially if you focus on doing stair work regularly and with good form.

## POOL:

- DEEP-WATER INTERVALS: medium-intensity level        20 minutes
  (See Exercises 1 to 4, pages 158 to 163.)

- DEEP WATERPOWER: all                                30 reps each
  (See Exercises 5 to 7 on pages 165 to 167.)

- KICK TRAINING: all                                  45 seconds each
  (See Exercises 8 to 11, pages 168 to 171.)

- GAIT TRAINING: all                                  1 minute each
  (See Exercises 12 to 14, pages 173 to 176.
  Wear a flotation belt the first few times
  you try bouncing, Exercise 14.)

- STRETCHING: curl and stretch, hamstring stretch,
  body swing                                          30 seconds each
  (See Exercises 15 to 17, pages 177 to 178.)
  quad stretch with strap or on step                  3 x 30 seconds
  (See Exercise 18 on page 179 and Exercise 3B on page 205.)

- WATERPOWER WORKOUT EXERCISES: all                   10 to 20 reps
                                                       with belt
  (See Exercises 21 to 26 on pages 181 to 184.
  Running, **with belt**, low- to moderate-intensity program
  (See Exercise 27 on pages 185 to 186.)              2 to 10 minutes

- LOWER EXTREMITY EXERCISES: all                       20 to 30 reps
  (See Exercises 28 to 34 on pages 189-195. Use a buoyancy
  cuff on Exercises 30 and 31. Reposition the step to shallower
  water for increased gravity to simulate step work on land.)

## LAND:

- NON-WEIGHTBEARING EXERCISES: all
  (See Exercises 1 and 5 to 11 on pages 202,            20 reps
  203, and 208 to 212.)

hamstring stretch, quad stretch, gastroc stretch    3 x 30 seconds
      (See Exercises 2 to 4 on pages 203 to 206.)

- WEIGHTBEARING EXERCISES: hamstring curls (both legs)    20 reps each
  toe raises, single leg stance
        (See Exercises 12 to14, page 213.)
- FUNCTIONAL EXERCISES: wall slides (limited painfree    10 reps each
  ROM) step-ups (four-inch only), mini-squats
        (See Exercises 16, 18, and 21, pages 214 to 216, and 218.)
- RESISTANCE EXERCISES: terminal knee extension    10 reps
  with Thera-band, quad extension with Thera-Band,
  hamstring curl with Thera-Band
        (See Exercises 22 to 24, pages 219 to 220.)
- BICYCLING: Stationary or recumbent bike    10 to 20 minutes,
  0 tension

## Phase Three

By now you'll be performing your ADLs without discomfort. You may still be experiencing stiffness, but your pain will be subsiding and minimal. During Phase Three you'll find you can accomplish more challenging functional activities, such as climbing a flight of stairs with a reciprocal pattern, rising from a lower chair, and squatting to a deeper position. Descending stairs may still be difficult, but don't worry—that's normal. Fine-tuning your normal pattern for going down stairs will be one of the most challenging of the last goals you'll accomplish. Even if you're not ready to reciprocate a full flight of stairs yet, try to reciprocate the first two steps as you go upstairs and the last two as you come down stairs. In the pool, you'll increase your intensity and reps and you'll remove your flotation belt unless it's needed due to pain. On land, you'll add most of the functional and resistance exercises. **Do not perform Exercise 20, single leg wall slides.**

## POOL:

- DEEP-WATER INTERVALS: high-intensity level                20 minutes
     (See Exercises 1 to 4, pages 158 to 164.)
- DEEP WATERPOWER: all                                      30 to 50 reps each
     (See Exercises 5 to 7 on pages 165 to 167.)
- KICK TRAINING: all                                        1 minute each
     (See Exercises 8 to 11, pages 168 to 171.
     Increase speed the last 30 seconds.)
- GAIT TRAINING: all                                        1 minute each
     (See Exercises 12 to 14 on pages 173 to 176. )
- STRETCHING: all                                           30 seconds each
     (See Exercises 15 to 20, pages 177 to 180.)
- WATERPOWER WORKOUT EXERCISES: all                         20 to 30 reps,
                                                            no belt
     (See Exercises 21 to 26 on pages 181 to 184.)
     running, no belt, moderate- to high-intensity program
                                                            10 to 15 minutes
     (See Exercise 27, pages 185 to 187.)
- LOWER EXTREMITY EXERCISES: all                            30 reps each
     (See Exercises 28 to 34, pages 189 to 195. Use a buoyancy
     cuff on Exercises 30 and 31. Reposition the step to shallower
     water for increased gravity to simulate land stepping.)

## LAND:

- NON-WEIGHTBEARING EXERCISES: all
     (See Exercises 1 and 5 to 11 on pages 202,        3 x 10 reps
     203, and 208 to 212.)
     hamstring stretch, quad stretch, gastroc stretch  3 x 30 seconds
     (See Exercises 2 to 4 on pages 203 to 206.)
- WEIGHTBEARING EXERCISES: all                         3 x 10 reps each
     (See Exercises 12 to 15 on pages 213 to 214.)
- FUNCTIONAL EXERCISES: wall slides, good mornings   20 to 30 reps
     step-ups, side step-ups, mini-squats
     (See Exercises 16 to19 and 21 on pages 214 to 218.
     Wall slide to 90 degrees, use a six-inch step on step-ups.)

- RESISTANCE EXERCISES: all              3 x 10 reps

                                                      2 to 3 x 10 reps

       (See Exercises 22 to 25, pages 219 to 221.)
- BICYCLING: stationary or recumbent bike      20 to 30 minutes, minimal tension

## YOUR MAINTENANCE PROGRAM

You're probably breathing a huge sigh of relief now that you've completed all three phases of your knee rehabilitation. Yet in spite of all the work you've already put into your healing knee, the work cannot stop here. You need to continue exercising for the rest of your life. Don't panic; you don't need to work at the same frequency of five times a week—three to four times a week should be fine. If you feel dysfunction creeping into your knee from lack of exercise, you can always resume the full-fledged program. Take charge of your knee: keep it strong and functioning smoothly so it can serve you for many years, if not an entire lifetime.

# GLOSSARY

**abduct**—to move a body part away from the midline of the body.

**abduction**—movement away from the midline of the body.

**active motion exercises**—exercises that require an active muscular contraction and movement at the joints.

**acute**—injury of recent onset.

**adduct**—moving toward the midline of the body.

**adduction**—movement toward the midline of the body.

**adhesions**—scar tissue formed by the body following injury or surgery.

**ADLs**—activities of daily living.

**allograft**—a tissue transferred between genetically dissimilar members of the same species.

**analgesic**—a drug that reduces pain.

**anesthesia**—a drug agent that causes the loss of sensation or consciousness.

**anesthesiologist**—a medical doctor who is certified as a specialist in the administration of anesthesia.

**antalgic gait**—walking with a limp because of pain.

**anterior**—pertaining to the front of a structure.

**anterior horn**—the front half of both the medial and lateral compartments of the knee joint.

**antipyretic**—a drug that lowers a fever.

**arthro**—Latin for "joint."

**arthroscope**—a pencil-thin surgical instrument that allows the surgeon to view inside the joint by way of a miniature video system and to operate on the interior of the joint.

**arthroscopy**—any surgical procedure that uses the arthroscope.

**articular cartilage**—also known as hyaline cartilage, it is the smooth thin layer that covers the ends of bones and protects the bones against impacting forces; the body's natural shock absorbers.

**aspirate**—to remove fluids from a cavity of the body.

**atelectasis**—a collapse of the small airways in the lungs, often causing fever after surgery.

**atrophy**—the shrinking in size of muscle tissue.

**autograft**—a tissue removed from one site and placed in another within the same individual.

**autoimmune disease**—when the body reacts against one of its own parts as if it were foreign. Rheumatoid arthritis is an autoimmune disease.

**avascular necrosis**—the loss of blood supply to the bone, which results in the death of the bone.

**avulsion fracture**—actually a ligament injury, when the ligament tears away from a bone pulling a bony piece of its anchoring site with it.

**bursa**—the fluid-containing sacs that provide cushioning around joints.

**bursitis**—inflammation of any of the bursa.

**chemical genomics**—the use of chemicals to fight the genetic breakdown that causes disease.

**chondral**—pertaining to the cartilage.

**chronic**—persisting over a long period of time.

**collagen**—a key protein composing bone, cartilage, tendons, and other tissues. In its most familiar form, collagen appears as a household product, gelatin.

**congenital**—present at birth.

**contracture**—a persistent constriction of the tissues, usually a muscle or joint capsule.

**contraindications**—things you should not do for a particular condition.

**crepitus**—creaking or crackling sound or sensation when moving a joint, a muscle, or a tendon.

**CT scan**—Computerized axial tomography, a three-dimensional X ray that is 100 times more sensitive than an ordinary X ray.

**deep vein thrombosis (DVT)**—a blood clot within a vein.

**displaced fracture**—a break in a bone where the pieces have pulled apart.

**distend**—to enlarge a space in the body by filling it with fluid.

**electrocardiogram (EKG)**—a test to monitor the electrical activity of the heart.

**embolism**—a blood clot that travels from one location to another within the body.

**ethernet**—a cable for transmitting information between networked, or linked, computers.

**extension**—straightening of a joint.

**fascia**—bands of fibrous tissues throughout the body that surround muscles.

**femur**—the thigh bone, the largest bone in the body.

**fibrocartilage**—the rubbery cartilage that composes the ears and the nose.

**flexion**—bending a joint.

**fracture**—a break or crack in a bone or cartilage.

**fulcrum**—the support or point of support on which a lever turns in raising or moving something.

**genome**—refers to the unique genetic information contained in the body's cells.

**Gerdy's tubercle**—the prominence of bone above and to the lateral side of the tibial tuberosity. Often used as a reference point, this is where the iliotibial band attaches.

**hyaline cartilage**—synonymous with articular cartilage; the shock-absorbing surfaces on the ends of bones.

**hyperextend**—straightening of a joint beyond the normal range of motion.

**hyperflex**—bending of a joint beyond the normal range of motion.

**ice massage**—applying ice to an injured area in a massaging manner to promote healing, achieve vaso-constriction, and control swelling.

**imaging studies**—all diagnostic studies that involve images, such as X rays, MRIs, CT Scans, ultra-sound, and mammograms.

**incentive spirometer**—a device given to a postsurgical patient that motivates him or her to breathe deeply. Visual feedback shows the depth and strength of each breath.

**inferior pole of the patella**—the lowest point of the patella, close to the tibia (shin bone).

**in-patient**—a patient who spends more than twenty-four hours in the hospital.

**internist**—a medical doctor certified in internal medicine.

**isokinetic exercise**—exercise that is variable and based upon the patient's strength. As the patient pushes harder, the resistance increases proportionately.

**isometric exercise**—exercise that does not involve any movement of the joint or limb; a fixed muscular contraction.

**IV**—intravenous fluids given to supply nutrients the body needs.

**kinesthetic sense**—the ability to perceive the position or angle of your joints without viewing them.

**knock-kneed**—deformity in which the knees are close together with increased space between the ankles.

**lateral**—pertaining to the area that is furthest from the midline of the body; the side or outer surface.

**lavage**—flushing out corrosive joint fluid with clear saline solution.

**level**—the brightness or darkness in an imaging study.

**ligaments**—strong, fibrous tissues that link bones at a joint.

**loose bodies**—fragments, usually of cartilage or bone, inside the joint.

**lymphatic system**—a body-wide drainage system for all fluids except blood. Where the blood uses the vascular system of arteries and veins, all other fluids are moved throughout the body within the lymphatic system.

**malleolus**—the prominence of bones on either side of the ankle. The medial malleolus is part of the tibia and the lateral malleolus is part of the fibula.

**medial**—pertaining to the area that is closest to the midline of the body; the middle or inner surface.

**medial collateral ligament**—the tough, fibrous connective tissue that runs down the medial aspect of the knee.

**meniscal cyst**—a soft, spongy growth on either the medial or lateral side of the knee; a collection of fluids from inside the knee joint due to a horizontal tear in the meniscus.

**menisci**—the plural of meniscus.

**meniscus**—the shock-absorbing, disk-like cartilage inside the knee joint.

**MRI**—magnetic resonance imaging. A diagnostic technology that uses a superconducting magnet and a computer precisely to display soft tissue and bone that is not apparent on an X ray.

**myofascial release**—a deep massage technique to release any constricted muscles, tendons, or fascia.

**non-displaced fracture**—a break in a bone where the pieces have not pulled apart.

**Nsaids**—non-steroidal anti-inflammatory drugs.

**orthopedist**—a medical doctor who is a specialist in treating disorders of the bones, muscles, joints, ligaments, tendons, and other parts of the musculoskeletal system.

**osteophytes**—spurs, or calcified outcroppings of bone.

**osteoporosis**—a loss of calcium and bone density, usually associated with aging.

**outpatient**—a patient who spends less than twenty-four hours in the hospital.

**overuse injuries**—injuries caused from doing too much of a single, repetitive movement.

**PACS**—Picture Archiving and Communications System, a digital system used for interpreting, storing, and transmitting filmless, imaging studies.

**palpate**—to examine by the sense of touch.

**patellar tendon**—the tendon that attaches the bottom of the kneecap to the tibia.

**patellofemoral joint**—the portion of the knee joint where, upon flexion or extension, the patella slides through the groove in the femur called the trochlea.

**pathognomonic**—specific to one thing only.

**peroneal nerve**—the nerve that supplies voluntary function of the toe and ankle extension.

**pes anserinus tendon**—the tendon of the semitendinosis muscle (one of the hamstrings), which at its attachment on the medial side of the tibia is similar to a goose's foot in appearance.

**placebo**—a medicine given merely to please the patient, but containing no true medicinal properties.

**popliteal artery**—continuation of the femoral artery as it runs behind the knee.

**popliteal tendon**—the tendon that attaches the popliteus muscle to the back of the femur. This tendon runs directly through the lateral meniscus.

**posterior**—pertaining to the back of a structure, to the rear.

**posterior horn**—the back half of both the medial and lateral compartments of the knee.

**prehab**—rehabilitation done prior to surgery.

**pre-op**—pre-operative, as in pre-op procedures and pre-op holding room.

**pre-patella bursa**—the bursal sac located in front of the kneecap to cushion the patella when kneeling.

**pronate**—to roll the foot inward.

**pronation**—complex motion of the foot that produces a flattening of the arch.

**prophylactic**—protecting or defending from disease; a preventive measure or drug.

**pseudo-laxity**—a condition in which the ligaments feel stretched out and the joint feels unstable, but no ligament injury has occurred. This condition occurs because the distance between bones decreases as the cartilage between the bones diminishes.

**pulmonary embolism**—a blood clot that lodges in the lungs.

**quadriceps**—the four muscles that run down the front of the thigh, causing hip flexion and knee extension.

**quadriceps tendon**—the tendon that attaches the quadriceps muscles to the top of the kneecap.

**radiologist**—a medical doctor who is a certified specialist in the interpretation of imaging studies, such as X rays, MRIs, and CT scans.

**reciprocate stairs**—to place one foot on a stair, then the opposite foot on the next stair above, and to continue alternating in this manner.

**red-red zone**—the outer one-third of a meniscus, so named because it is nourished through the blood supply from the knee joint capsule.

**red-white zone**—the middle one-third of a meniscus. It receives half of its nourishment from blood circulation and half from the sponge-like system of the joint fluids.

**rehabilitation**—reconditioning of the musculoskeletal system to restore maximum function.

**rheumatologist**—a medical doctor who is a certified specialist in rheumatological diseases, including rheumatoid arthritis, lupus, osteoarthritis, and fibromyalgia.

**rounds**—the common phrase for a doctor's visits to his patients in the hospital following surgery.

**rupture**—a complete tear of a body's structure, often a ligament or tendon.

**saline solution**—salt water.

**sclerosis**—a uneven hardening of the bone due to unequal weight-bearing in a joint.

**scull**—the use of the hands when submerged in water to correctly position or move the body.

**sesamoid bone**—a small round bone found in tendons and some muscles with the function of increasing the capability of a joint by improving the angle of approach of the tendon into its insertion. The patella is the largest sesamoid bone in the body.

**spur**—an abnormal bone growth at the edge of joints.

**stenosis**—narrowing of a canal or opening, often applied to a narrowing of the various openings in the vertebrae that pinch the nerves.

**subchondral bone**—the bone directly beneath the hyaline or articular cartilage.

**subcutaneous**—beneath the skin.

**superficial**—close to the surface.

**supinate**—to roll outward.

**supination**—complex motion of the foot that produces an increase in the arch.

**supine**—lying on the back, face up.

**synovectomy**—the removal of a portion or all of the inflamed lining of a joint.

**synovial fluid**—the lubricating fluid within the joints.

**synovium**—the lining of a joint.

**synovial lining**—synonymous with synovium, the lining of a joint.

**tendinitis**—inflammation of a tendon.

**tendons**—the fibrous cords of connective tissue that attach muscles to bones.

**Thera-Bands**—latex bands used for resistance exercises.

**tibial plateau**—the top of the tibia that is coated with hyaline cartilage.

**trochlea**—a part of the knee joint; the groove in the femur or thigh bone where the patella glides when the knee is bent or straightened.

**vascular**—pertaining to the blood vessels.

**vasoconstriction**—narrowing of the blood vessels resulting in a reduction of blood flow.

**vasodilation**—enlargement of the blood vessels resulting in increased blood flow.

**vastus medialis oblique**—the most medial of the four quadricips muscles; the muscle most able to hold the patella in its correct tracking alignment.

**VMO**—see vastus medialis oblique muscle.

**white-white zone**—the innermost and thinnest one-third of the wedge-shaped meniscus. It depends solely on joint fluid for its nourishment.

**window**—the contrast between light and dark in a grayscale imaging study.

**X ray**—electromagnetic radiation that passes through the body to create a picture of the dense tissues of the body, such as bone.

# APPENDIX

The following is a list of products that appeared in the text.

**AquaJogger**—the most easily obtained floatation belt, since it is carried by most sporting good stores. This belt is best when used by people with small waists. If someone large of girth wears it, the flotation is all at the back of the body with only a strap across the front, which makes balance more difficult.

***The Complete Waterpower Workout Book***—Lynda Huey's bestselling water exercise book.

**HAN Wet Belt**—the favorite belt of CompletePT's pool director, Pattie O'Leary. This two-piece belt provides equal buoyancy around the entire body, and also offers support for those with lower-back complaints.

**Hydro-Fit Cuffs**—buoyancy cuffs which, when used on ankles, help create increased range of motion for knees during quad extension and hamstring curls.

**Hydro-Tone Belt and Boot**—one of the most buoyant of the belts, but best used by tall people since its width at the front can be uncomfortable, particularly for short women who complain of it pressing on their ribcages and chests. A powerful resistance piece for increased leg strength.

**Laminated Knee Therapy Pool Program card**—a two-sided exercise card with the photos from this book to guide you poolside.

**Lynda Huey's Waterpower Workout video**—a one-hour pool class with beautiful underwater shots of Deep Waterpower, Stretching, Kick Training, Waterpower, Upper body and lower body exercises.

**Thermo-X Shirt**—pullover, fleece-lined shirt for warmth; comes in short-sleeves or long-sleeves.

**Tru-Fit**—freezable gel packs that fit into a fabric holder with velcro straps. Gel packs can also be micro-waved for contrasting heat treatment.

**Waterpower Workout Tether**—stretching tubing plus canvas fabric provide the right amount of "give" for running in place in shallow water. Tethering to the side of the pool lifts the body into proper form during deep-water intervals.

**Wave Belt**—one of the least buoyant of belts, but narrow at the front, so this belt is good for short people with a normal or greater amount of body fat. The Wave Belt is also excellent as a second belt on top of either the Hydro-Tone or HAN Wet Belt for people who need increased buoyancy.

**Wet Shirt**—a neoprene, zip-up, short-sleeve shirt for additional warmth.

**Wet Sweat Belt**—Lynda Huey's favorite belt. It provides enough buoyancy for many athletes while also offering a narrow attachment at the front—a bonus for those who are short.

All of these items can be ordered from:
Huey's Athletic Network
800/909-0300
310/829-5622
www.lahuey.com

### Robert Klapper, M.D.

Robert Klapper was born and raised in Queens, New York. He received his undergraduate degree in art history from Columbia University in New York, then entered Columbia's College of Physicians and Surgeons where he specialized in orthpedic surgery. An internship at Cedars-Sinai Medical Center in Los Angeles was followed by a residency at the Hospital for Special Surgery in New York, then a fellowship in arthritis and implant surgery at the Kerlan-Jobe Clinic in Los Angeles. He is currently Clinical Chief of Orthopedics at Cedars-Sinai Medical Center in Los Angeles. He takes pride in being a surgeon, an inventor with six patents for surgical tools, an award-winning sculptor, and a surfer. He lives in Encino, California, with his wife.

### Lynda Huey

Lynda Huey was born and raised in northern California where she received her bachelor's and master's degrees from San Jose State University. She taught and coached at California Polytechnic State University, Oberlin College, Los Angeles City College, Santa Monica College, and UCLA. She moved to southern California in 1975 for competition in track and field and beach volleyball and to be near Wilt Chamberlain, her longtime companion. Her autobiography, *A Running Start: An Athlete, A Woman* was published in 1976; her first water exercise book, *The Waterpower Workout* was published in 1986. Her third book, *The Complete Waterpower Workout Book,* published in 1993, is in its ninth printing and has been translated into German and Spanish. In 1999 she opened *CompletePT* Pool & Land Physical Therapy in Los Angeles. Lynda is a world-renowned lecturer and leader in the water exercise and therapy industry. She lives in Santa Monica, California.

### Contributor Tanya Moran-Dougherty, MPT

Tanya Moran-Dougherty, MPT, contributed the land exercises to Chapters 1 and 11 and offered guidance on designing programs in Chapters 8 and 14. She was born and raised in Allentown, Pennsylvania. She received her undergraduate degree in exercise physiology from Pennsylvania State University. Her post-graduate work in physical therapy was completed at Temple University in Philadelphia. Tanya has been the clinical director for Complete PT since 2000. She lives in Redondo Beach, California, with her husband, Brian.

# INDEX